I Did It, You Can Too!

I Did It, You Can Too!

How I Lost 70lbs and Became a Fitness Coach

James Mullins

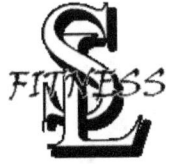

Semper Liberi Fitness
4802 Orchard St
South Charleston, WV 25309
www.slf.fit

Printed in the United States of America

Publisher's Cataloging-in-Publication data
Mullins, James.
I Did It, You Can Too: How I Lost 70lbs and Became A Fitness Coach
James Mullins

Second Edition

In memory of my father,

who teaches me, even now.

Acknowledgements

Throughout this book, I have had the opportunity to share many different thoughts about how this book came to exist and some of the people who allowed this journey to take place. There are others who I want to take a moment to thank and acknowledge that helped me with this creation process.

First, my wonderful wife. She always allows me to be myself and supports and idea I may have or any way that I wish to express myself. Without her, I would not I would not have the confidence to share my thoughts with the world.

I also want to thank everyone in my family and in the community where I grew up. I felt an incredible amount of love growing up, and I always felt that I had a supportive environment. Many things have changed since I moved away, but I developed great values that I hold dear from being raised in an area where helping others, and caring was important. I would not have wanted to grow up anywhere else in the world.

I want to thank those involved in our mastermind group. Their help and input were instrumental in making this available to you.

Lastly, thanks to everyone that has played a part in my career and physical development. I have had the benefit of many great coaches, teachers, supervisors, and mentors throughout my life and each of them have played a part in developing me so that I could accomplish this task.

These great people have all had a positive impact and helped influence my life. I am grateful for them all and I am glad that I have been able to share this journey with you. I hope that I have a positive influence in your life similarly to those who have influenced mine. Thanks, James

Preface

Everyone has their own story to tell. Everyone has dealt with their own struggles, their own fear, and their own obstacles. We each have many different events and people who impact and effect our lives. What do we do with these events, and how can we use them to help ourselves grow and become better?

This is what I want to share with you. How to use events and circumstances in your life to help yourself and others grow and embrace the freedom that life has to offer. I know there are others out there who feel the way I use to feel and share the same limiting beliefs and doubts that I use to.

I use to feel chained down. Chained to a body that was overweight, tired, and lacking energy. Chained to a job where I felt like I was not making a difference or having an impact. Chained to a lifestyle where I felt like I was not in control of my goals or the outcome of my life.

I found a way out! I found the confidence, self-esteem, and personal belief to chase my own potential and begin a journey to improve myself physically, mentally, and emotionally each day.

I want to share my journey with you. I want you to know the mistakes I made so you can avoid them. I want you to have tools and resources available so that you can begin your own journey of self-discovery, physical freedom, and personal growth without the trial and error that I went through.

I have seen the benefits of changing your life by building your body, confidence, and self-esteem and the impact it can have in everything you do. I want you to be able to take this same journey.

My mission since the inception of my company has been to offer a positive and supportive environment for others who want to become healthy and fit, and this book is an extension of that.

I want my story to help you build confidence, self esteem, and knowledge. I want you to feel like you can do anything and break down any limiting beliefs and fears that you have and reach for the best that you can be.

I want you to know there is someone out there like you who went through the same struggles. The goal of sharing my story here is to help you achieve your goals in life. I want to help you develop yourself both mentally and physically and allow you to begin to gain the confidence you need to succeed and live the life of your dreams.

Introduction

Before we get into the nuts and bolts of the book, I want to explain to you just exactly what this book is intended to be and how it may help you. I know your time is very important, and I want you to be sure that this is for you before you make the investment of reading it.

If you are someone who wants to lose weight or start your own business, then this is a book for you. If you were looking for a fitness program that you will enjoy and want some advice from someone who has tried many, then this book is for you. If you feel like you can do more and that you are destined to great things but don't know where to begin then this book is definitely for you.

This book is not going to be a literary masterpiece, so if you are looking for great writing, then this is not for you. I am not a writer. I am just a normal person trying to share stories and experiences and share them in a simple and easy to understand way.

This book is not, a step by step fitness solution to solve all of your weight loss or health problems. It also is not a business book with step by step instructions on how to build each step of a successful business.

The goal, however, is by the end of the book for you to have the available resources and confidence to begin both building the body you want and the business you want.

You see I want to inspire others to do what they love and have confidence in themselves. I want others to have the freedom that comes from being fit and healthy and owning your own business. I think the best way for me to do this is to share my own experiences with others and let them see someone just like them who started with limited resources and many doubters. Someone who was surrounded with limiting beliefs about the possibility of success and how I learned and grew along that journey.

Whether you want to start a successful business or build the body you want, you will find some insight and ideas of how to begin. I will provide you with the resources and input I have gathered from my own journey and share some of my mistakes along the way.

This is kind of like two books in one. It is a bit of an autobiography chronicling the fitness portion of my life and how it ties into my career and personal life. A portion is going to be about ways you can learn and utilize the different programs I tried and things you can take away from my experiences in those programs. And the second part is the actual programs themselves which you can use as a beginner guide to fitness.

I want you to be able to use this book as a starter guide about how to get in shape and learn from my experiences so you have an easier path. However, I didn't go about my experience in a nice linear path so it is not set up as a nice linear program. I have included small sample workout programs similar to the types of programs I used. These are the things that allowed me to develop along the way, and I want to share a portion so you can experience some of the many different types of program and styles available to get fit and healthy.

I don't want you to go through the trial and error of finding the specific type of fitness program that you will enjoy. I don't want you to have to spend months trying a program only to find that it doesn't suit you and then quit without getting the results you want. I want you to have a fitness sampler that allows you to see a portion of many types of fitness programs so that you can find what works best for you.

Any fitness chapter in this book can be taken out and made into its own separate book with much more information and program knowledge added to make a structured program with that style or type of training.

At some point I may decide to do just that and write my strength and conditioning manual, cross training manual, running manual, etc. but that is not what this is intended to be. There are many other books out there if you want to read in depth about anything I cover in this book.

I want this book to be about my journey and the many different stops along the way and how that journey can help you. I want to give you a portion of each program I tried so you can sample a variety of fitness types and decide which one is right for you.

I have put a lot of time and effort into the portions of the programs that are included, and they are great beginner programs that you will get huge benefits from. You will see progress after using them, and they will get you on a path to losing weight and being healthy. They are not the only aspects of these programs that I used to see results they are only part of a longer program.

If you want more in-depth information or your own personalized program, then our coaching program delivers that, and we would be glad to help you reach your goals. This book is just a guideline of how I progressed through my fitness journey.

I want to share that journey with you. I want you to know where I came from and what steps I have taken to get to where I am now. I want this book to be two things that give you equal value in each.

I want this book to be a tool you can utilize as a guide to begin to make changes to your body and mind. I want you to be able to take the workouts and nutritional information and utilize it to begin your path to the physique you dream of.

With the included information you will be able to begin a physical transformation and achieve your fitness goals. I know each program will work, and you can achieve your goals with them.

As I said these programs are a beginner's portion to give you a sampler of fitness so you can choose your main course. However, each program can be repeated for several cycles allowing you to progress from the beginner level and see results.

A basic transformation program and the ones designed for this book are structured for 12-week blocks. However, due to the many different types of programs included I was only able to include a portion of the 12-week block. You can extend any program in this book to 12 weeks. Since the programs are not structured for the long term make sure that you take an active recovery/deload week between cycles of the program to ensure you continue to progress.

This book will give you the tools to succeed, but if you want or need more help I have many resources available for free at www.slf.fit/free to help you. If that isn't enough and you still need help, then we will gladly assist you in achieving your goal. Just check out the coaching information at www.slf.fit/coaching.

My main objective with this book is to make sure you have all of the tools and resources you need to move toward your goals. I want to provide you with the resources you need to succeed so that moving forward, ability and knowledge, will not be a roadblock.

The second objective I want this book to accomplish is to be an inspiration to anyone who reads it. I want you to know that I don't think of my story as some great, inspirational tale. There are many other people who have accomplished much more at a much greater disadvantage than I ever faced.

I have drawn my own inspiration from many of these very people, and I don't want anyone to think that I am comparing myself to any of these truly inspiring individuals. However, I do think my story is inspiring in its own way. I think everyone has their own story to tell and each story will resonate and inspire someone.

As I said, my second goal is to inspire each person that reads this in some small way. I want you to see how similar we are showing you that with the proper guidance and determination that you too can achieve any goal you chose.

I have some questions for you included throughout the book so that you can reflect and see how you and I may have similar backgrounds or experiences. I want you to understand that none of the things I talk about or that you hope to achieve are out of your reach. Hopefully, afterward, you will begin your own journey and create your own story that inspires others.

1

Where did you grow up?

"There are things about growing up in a small town that you can't necessarily quantify."

- Brandon Routh

Are you from a small town? What obstacles did you run into because of where you grew up? Do you think you missed out on anything? Did you have the options and educational opportunities available to be fit and healthy?

Well, let's look at these questions and reflect on them as we go. How do we relate to one another? Did we have similar obstacles growing up? The good news is, as you will soon see, it doesn't matter where you are from or what your past obstacles were. You can take the steps to move forward, learn, and grow.

I grew up in a small town, a really small town. It was a small rural area with nothing to do and nothing worthy of note except our high school (which is now closed by the way). There was a small two lane road, and railroad tracks and that was about it.

The nearest Wal-Mart, hospital and County Seat were 25 minutes away. Everything in our area meant that a commute was involved and until you could drive there was nothing to do and nowhere to do it. You were stuck at home. And this was back before the internet. We didn't have city water. I didn't have paved roads to skate on or a park to play in. Our area didn't have high-speed internet until around 2010.

I would continue to describe to you just how boring things were, but it was so bad that the adjectives and visualizations are beyond my capabilities as a writer. Now don't get me wrong, I loved where I grew up. I was lucky enough to be surrounded by family and friends who loved me, and I am very fortunate to have had those wonderful people to help shape my life. Some would look at a small town and say that it left no chance for opportunity. While this may be true in some ways, it did allow for a very personal and nurturing environment.

What was your community like growing up? Did you have a fitness center? Did you know anyone who was involved in health or fitness? What was your high school like and how did that experience shape you?

Our high school was a junior high/high school grades 7-12 with an enrollment of around 350 students. This allowed for a very small and individualized approach to our education. It also allowed us to form real relationships with our teachers, classmates, and faculty. Our school was our community.

Since the school was the main focus of the community, everything revolved around those activities. There were no other opportunities to meet people, no other social gatherings, and no other activities other than those made available by the school.

This lack of available social activities and the inability to interact with the outside world meant that the only means of release was sports. So as a youth I was involved in basketball and baseball (our school was too small for a football team). My parents really enjoyed my participation in sports and the social gatherings that it included so they always kept me involved. It was a good idea since I was what they called a" husky" child and would have been in even worse physical condition if not for sports.

What social opportunities did you have? How did they influence your health and fitness? How would things have been different if you had the same social opportunities that technology has made available now?

Socialization and community interaction were very important and sports provided that for everyone in our area. The other events in the area that allowed people to socialize and communicate were church and family gatherings. This left sports as the only social event that focused on fitness while both church and family events usually had a major focus on food.

Being from a rural are like this, we always had great food which was a major factor in my being overweight during childhood. I have always enjoyed eating and food was always something that was readily available. Anytime you went to anyone's home they would always offer you wonderful food. Rural staples like gravy and biscuits, pancakes, eggs, sausage, pinto beans, cornbread, chicken n dumplings, fried chicken, fried potatoes, and many other great foods. One thing is for sure, everyone always made you feel welcome by offering you food.

What foods did you love growing up? How have your tastes changed? Are you more open to trying new things now than you were when you were younger?

Unfortunately, none of these foods we enjoyed growing up were the healthiest options. You see living in such a small rural area meant that we had very few people who talked about health and nutrition. At our gatherings, everyone always brought a dish of food, but no one really understood or discussed the benefits of being active and playing games during these events. We didn't have a fitness center, nor do I remember anyone really talking about eating healthy or being fit.

Once in high school, you would hear more focus on the importance of being in shape for sports, but there were never any discussions about nutrition and improving athletic performance with diet or exercise. The sport was the exercise, and it was how we managed to stay in healthy.

Even though we had sports to help us stay fit, our eating habits didn't change. We still attended the same social gatherings and enjoyed the same unhealthy foods. Sports allowed us to remain healthy and fit, but there were no opportunities for fitness besides sports participation.

We didn't have a weight room or a strength coach so there was never anyone to emphasize the importance of fitness for athletics or health. This has led me to understand how the obesity rate has risen the way it has and how a lack of education and awareness has played a major part in our nation's rising health issues. No one in our area knew the ramifications that could arise from poor eating habits and lack of exercise so health was not a major concern.

So my health and fitness levels actually improved in high school with the increased activity in athletics, and I was at what I now call my fat, skinny weight of 180lbs. I say this because even though I was thin, I had no noticeable muscle mass. This is the weight I maintained throughout high school until I quit playing basketball my senior year.

What was your activity level like in high school? Were you more active or less active than you are now? What activities did you enjoy then and is there a way you can participate in them now?

2

Life After Sports

"An unfortunate thing about this world is that the good habits are much easier to give up than the bad ones." - W. Somerset Maugham

I quit playing sports in my senior year of high school. I was never someone driven by the competition of sports and I did not feel a link to my sports participation and self-image. I played sports because I enjoyed playing and because I liked to compete. This was not the mentality of those in our community. Everyone in the community believed that sports were the most important focus.

Since I was not driven by sports success, once I found other interests, I stepped away from the participation. I never enjoyed practice or games, and the importance placed on them. I always felt forced to do something that I previously did for enjoyment. I did still enjoy the actual sports, so I would occasionally play as a hobby but not competitively in the school system.

Even though I still played sports on occasion, it was not often enough to help keep me fit and healthy. Since I was poorly educated about diet and nutrition, I continued to eat like I was a teenager playing sports. This meant that I was constantly eating pizza, Oreo cookies, powdered doughnuts, peanut butter & jelly, strawberry milk, and fast food. I was an eating machine.

Did your eating habits change after high school? How about your activity levels? What major changes did you have after graduating?

I would go through a package of Oreos in two days, a 24 pack of soda in three, and a loaf of bread in four. I would wake up in the middle of the night and drink a can of soda and then go back to bed. My parents said that I was eating them out of house and home and looking back on it, that may have been true.

I would go to the Olive Garden once every two weeks and if they had the never ending pasta I could go through several bowls with salad and bread sticks. The worst though was the soda. My dad would buy 24 packs. I have always consumed a lot of fluids so they didn't last long at all. I have since estimated that I consumed around 1500-2000 calories a day just from the liquids I consumed.

The thing is, I didn't know I had a problem. I just ate, and everyone acted like it was normal because I had always been a big eater.

That may have been fine, had I continued to be as active as I was but without the activity, my body changed.

Without the activity of sports, and with my poor eating habits, I went from a lean 180lb basketball player to an overweight 250lb couch potato. I was constantly playing video games (which I also did as a teenager so that isn't an excuse) and eating. Neither my family or doctor approached me to discuss how I was changing.

I know that is a hard conversation to have, and I know that I probably wouldn't have listened to my family or friends, but it would have at least helped me acknowledge there was a problem. You think people who lack a filter and say harsh things are bad, but sometimes it can awaken you to a real issue.

I, however, continued to be in the dark. Now deep down, I knew I wasn't where I wanted to be. I remember a pool party I had before going to college, and I didn't take my shirt off during the party. Looking back, it was because I was unhappy with my body but at the time there wasn't anything that made me acknowledge this.

I knew that I was in poor shape. I was beginning to move more slowly, and being overweight was a struggle. At one point in time, I did become slightly more active but only because I was still around some of the friends that I played sports with, and we would still play occasionally in our free time.

My weight loss at this point was just a nice addition to something I enjoyed and not a realization of the need to change. But it was a small improvement, and I lost 25lbs. I was down from my top weight of 250 to around 225 just by being active, lifting weights with friends (our school finally got a weight room after I quit sports), and playing sports.

This change occurred while I was still living with my parents and still around the friends I had grown up with. I went to a community college for my Associate's Degree, and this allowed me to live at home and continue to be active with friends. I might have continued to lose weight and stay active but to get my Bachelor's Degree I had to transfer to a different school so, at this point, it was off to college.

I moved out of my parents' home, got married, got a job, and went to college. At this point, I weighed in around 220-225lbs, and I remained at that weight through most of my college years.

I had what I figure is the typical college experience where you don't have time to focus on your health, and you are busy with other things. Now, I have never been a drinker so I didn't go through that phase of college where I gained weight during my freshmen year and kept it on until after college. I just went to college overweight and remained overweight throughout.

Did you go to college? If so, what was your college experience like? Did you gain weight and struggle to stay in shape or did you play sports and stay active?

My college days were very busy. I had a full-time job and worked third shift on overnights several months throughout the year in addition to my class schedule. There were days where I was gone to school from 8:00 am until 9:00 pm, and I had to be at work at 10:00 pm. This meant that I had to sleep in my truck in between classes to get rest.

As you can tell, my schedule and lifestyle did not support a fitness routine. I didn't have any free time, but I still wanted to be active. This meant looking for ways to be active at home. My wife and I lived in a small one-bedroom apartment so what I did was buy an exercise bike, dumbbells, a bench, and a small doorway pull-up bar.

I don't know if I ever used the pull-up bar, and I don't really remember using the bench. I do remember riding the exercise bike and playing video games and thinking that was a fitness program that would make a difference.

Guess what, it didn't. I continued to stay at the same weight, and I lacked commitment, focus, and knowledge about how to get in shape. I continued my work in retail, going to college, and ignoring my physical problems.

Every now and then I would make a half-hearted attempt at weight training by using plans and programs from the bodybuilding magazines that I had grown to love as a teenager. This interest in weight training continued to grow and even though I still wasn't completely committed to a fitness program my interest in bodybuilding was continuing to grow.

3

Why I Love Bodybuilding

"The resistance that you fight physically in the gym and the resistance that you fight in life can only build a strong character." - Arnold Schwarzenegger

Aside from my previous participation in sports, I would attribute my venture into fitness to bodybuilding.

Since basketball was the sport I participated in the most during high school, and since my school didn't have a football team, this left me as a thin "skinny fat" teenager.

I only weighed 180lbs, but I had no muscle definition and no real strength. Without a weight room and a strength coach at our school, there was no emphasis on weight training.

I would have continued along the path of using sports to meet my fitness needs if not for a couple of family members who talked me into going to the gym. They were planning to join a gym and offered to let me tag along. Having a few girls talk about how much they liked muscular guys and how they thought that going to the gym was a great idea didn't hurt with motivation either.

So I went and after the first few times, I was hooked. I had times since when I stayed away from training due to time constraints and life issues but the love I have for lifting weights ignited then and has stayed with me. When I was younger, I didn't have the proper fitness knowledge or direction to see significant results, but I did find enjoyment in the actual process of lifting weights. I developed a love for the physical feeling and mental focus involved in weight training. The reasons that this passion grew can be attributed to bodybuilding.

Bodybuilding magazines were what led our trio to begin going to the gym. In our small town, it was the only resource (no internet back then, boy am I old) we had that mentioned strength training or muscle growth. These magazines were our window to the possibilities for the human physique. The magazines were the bridge between the action heroes was saw on television and in comic books and our real world.

We would take these magazines and use the programs as a guide. We would look at these mass monsters and dream of being built like them some day. We were misguided and untrained, but it did ignite a fire and love to train that I still have today.

Eventually, before I left my small town, we did get a gym. We still only had limited resources, so the magazine plans were our roadmap. The magazines did not focus as heavily on nutrition as they do now, and the pictures of food they included at the time were not that appealing. Since we were not well educated about the importance of nutrition and the meals didn't look appetizing (nothing like our fried potatoes and pinto beans anyway) we didn't follow any nutritional advice. Because we ignored nutrition, the magazines did nothing for our physique.

I continued to utilize magazines even after I moved away from home. They were my resource for fitness information and without the proper nutritional guidance I never saw results while using them.

All was not lost. As I said, I had developed a love for bodybuilding. Even when I was too busy to train, and while I went through my weight gain, I followed bodybuilding. I learned about the sport, the benefits, and the people.

Like every guy who has touched a weight, I began to admire Arnold Schwarzenegger and everything he accomplished. I wanted a physique like that. I wanted to be huge like the guys in these magazines.

I began to read about the legends of bodybuilding. I read about Lou Ferrigno, Sergio Oliva, Franco Columbo, Frank Zane, and Reg Park just to name a few. I started reading about the Olympia, Robert Kennedy, and Joe Weider. I became consumed with everything bodybuilding.

This love naturally led to their books. I read Arnold's books, the books published by the magazines, and any article or magazine I could get. I had many subscriptions to various bodybuilding magazines.

I wanted to build a body like these and I thought this was the training I needed to do it.

I want to share what I found in my time bodybuilding. I enjoy lifting weights. I would rather lift weights than do cardio. Lifting weight alone, won't get you the body in these magazines.

Let me elaborate. If you genuinely love to train and lift weights, then bodybuilding is an excellent way to shape and change your body.

However, you need time to do it. I went the bodybuilding route but time became an issue.

To be built like the professionals in the magazines, you need to be willing to put in great sacrifices and lots of time and effort. The professionals train for a living and the average person will have a hard time making that commitment.

You must be willing to put in an hour in the gym, perform cardio for the required time, and alter your diet drastically to look like a professional bodybuilder. While I enjoy the actual process of lifting weights, I do not want to make huge sacrifices and alter my lifestyle to look like a bodybuilder.

Another realization from all of the research and knowledge I gained from bodybuilding is that there are limits to genetics. I finally had enough knowledge and experience to realize that the men on the magazines I loved used pharmaceuticals to obtain their size.

Research by Natural Bodybuilder - Casey Butt shows that there are limitations to the natural amount of muscle mass a person can gain depending on their body type and size. I began to look at natural bodybuilders and see their limits compared to those who gained all of the publicity in the magazines.

All of this information led me to the realization that if I wanted to look like the legends, that I would need assistance. Once again this was another sacrifice I was not willing to make. Just to be clear, I have no problem with someone who decides to use steroids, HGH, or any other performance enhancing drug.

I am not concerned with the ethics of pharmaceuticals; I just don't think they should be done without proper supervision. I don't believe that anyone should risk their health to look or perform better. Until they are legal and administered by doctors, I'm all for the natural route.

So by now you have probably concluded that I was not the best "bodybuilder" since I was unwilling to make all of the sacrifices necessary to achieve success. I gave it a shot anyway, but I didn't see progress until after I used P90X to lose my body fat.

After I went through P90X and saw my transformation, I went back to the bodybuilding format. I still use it from time to time, and it is very similar to the hypertrophy training of a strength and conditioning program.

I saw decent results after revisiting but time has always been a concern for me while utilizing a bodybuilding program. I find it hard to schedule both a workout session and a cardio session, so I prefer a circuit training style program.

As I said, I love bodybuilding, I love lifting weights, and I enjoy the time it allows me to spend in the gym. But for me, it was to time intensive and my career requirements and other interests limit the time I have available to spend in the gym. I think bodybuilding is the best type of programming for adding muscle mass, and if you are willing to make the sacrifices, then you will enjoy it and see the rewards.

However, be realistic, understand the limits you and your body have, and realize that you can only get so far naturally. With that, I would suggest bodybuilding as the program to utilize as an ectomorph trying to gain mass. So if that is your goal get a program, and have fun!

4

My Life Changing Event

"Someone has to die in order that the rest of us should value life more."

\- Virginia Woolf

So we have touched on how I gained interest in bodybuilding. We discussed the love I have for weight training but let's back up a minute and take a look at some things that led to my physical transformation. Let's see how you might relate to my physical and emotional state when I realized that change was needed.

Have you ever come to a major realization that change was necessary? Has there ever been a major event in your life that made you stop and take inventory of your life? Have you ever lost someone dear to you? Have you had a health issue or injury?

Well, I had several events that made me reflect and look at things differently.

I was continuing with my overweight, overworked, and overstressed lifestyle. I had constant struggles like going to college, a crazy retail schedule, and no time for anything fun. I continued this routine and kept hoping life would get better. It didn't.

I was offered a promotion at work. I know, you must be thinking, isn't that better? Yeah, it was better, but that depends on your point of view. A job promotion also meant more responsibility and because it was moving to a salaried position from an hourly position it meant more time invested. It also meant that I seemed to be choosing retail as a career and not as a way to support myself during school.

A career promotion did allow my wife and me the ability to buy a house and have a better financial situation. It also meant that school was going to be the second focus for me. I had been in college for six years due to the limited class schedule that I had to take while working. I decided since the school was now an afterthought that I should reevaluate my plan.

Upon evaluation, I found that the classes I needed to get my Engineering Degree were only offered during the fall semester (our busiest time in the toy industry). I normally work 80-90 hrs. a week at this point in the year (fourth quarter, during the holiday season) and those hours are on the overnight shift. This led me to a very hard decision.

I decided to stop going to school and focus on my career. I know this seems like a poor decision, but I had absolutely no free time, and I was miserable. I enjoyed retail, and I knew I could make a career doing it. So I decided to quit college classes and focus on my job.

Neither of my parents went to college and just by working hard and advancing in my retail career I was already making more money than both of my parents as a retail supervisor. There were so many limited opportunities where I grew up that I was led to a limiting belief that I had achieved enough success and didn't need to worry about other career options.

Quitting school to pursue a management career did allow me to free up some time, and now once again I was beginning to think about fitness. Not health, just getting into shape and looking better. This is the point where I began looking for ways to be more active and talking to others at work who may be interested in doing the same.

Have you run into issues with finding time to work out? Are you completely overwhelmed leaving no time for fitness? Is there anything you can do to change your schedule to manage some time for fitness and health? Do you have anyone who might be interested in exercising with you?

While discussing fitness with others, I found a coworker who was also interested in getting in better shape. Both of us continued to put it off and look for ways to avoid the actual process. This is a trap that most people fall into. They keep talking about making a change but are not committed enough to go through with it. It is really easy to talk about change. It is also really easy to continue to search for resources and avoid taking action. This is what leads to some of the many types of procrastination like "Analysis Paralysis" and "Perfection Paralysis" that I discuss with clients.

That is exactly where we were, and I would have continued to talk about it and not take action if not for a life-changing event.

While home for Thanksgiving my father told me, he had lung cancer. It was the saddest I had ever seen him, and I could tell how hard it was for him to break that news to me. He told me about the diagnosis and that he was going to have surgery soon.

I had grown accustomed to news like this since my father had ill health for many years. My father smoked for more than 40 years and had some major health problems. He had heart and lung issues and was in the hospital frequently which meant that I spent a great deal of time around hospitals.

My father spent the last 20 years or so of his life with very limited physical abilities due to the unhealthy lifestyle he lived. Sadly, like many other people he did not know the choices he was making would have a negative impact until it was too late to make a change.

With the frequent health issues my father had and the time, I spent around him, you would think that I might have realized how important health and fitness were and would take a bigger interest in my own health.

Unfortunately, this isn't how things normally work out, and I hadn't begun to see how important health was. I still felt invincible, and I figured things would turn out as usual. I thought we would have another hospital stay, and he would recover without any problems. I always made sure that I was optimistic so my father would keep his spirits up during his hospital stay. So when he shared this information with me at Thanksgiving, I told him to stick to the doctor's plan, and we would hope for the best.

I didn't know it at the time, but this was the last Thanksgiving I would spend with him. He had surgery that December and even though we thought he was going to recover and make it home, he fell ill, and passed away.

Now when something like this happens in life, there are many different ways you can look at it and it has a huge effect on your life. I chose to be grateful. It wasn't an easy process to deal with, and my mother had a very difficult time, but I understood a few simple things that I want to share with you in hopes that they may help you during a time when you experience the loss of a loved one.

I looked at my father passing in several ways, but the biggest takeaway I had was how grateful I was to have had him as a father. I knew how he shaped me and how that contributed to everything I had done in my life.

I was saddened because I knew that I could not continue to share experiences with him and that he wasn't here to support or guide me anymore. But I knew that our universe is a vast place and with all of the circumstances and random chance occurrences that I was blessed to have had him as my father. I knew just how fortunate I was and how things had to align just right for these events to occur. This gave me a sense of peace.

It made me look at the whole ordeal with a different view. While I was sad, I started to feel more sadness for those around me instead of myself. I knew what an impact my father had on my life, and I had only spent 25 years with him. I felt sorry for those who had spent much more time with him than I had.

I thought about how much they must be hurting because if I was hurting as bad as I was and I was feeling this great loss based on the short time he had impacted my life, then those who had known him for 50+ years must be completely broken.

This realization allowed me to share many great stories and really connect with my family about how my father impacted them. It took a miserable experience and brought us all together. It allowed me to see that the best way of moving forward is to find a way to reframe your outlook on a situation. You can you make it into something positive. You can you grow from it. You can see how it has shaped you for the better and not how it has broken you moving forward.

It was the key event in my life, and it changed the way that I think about everything. It let me refocus, and I realized I need to look at my own life and be sure to get the best out of it.

I moved forward knowing that I would be successful with my new position and everything else I chose to pursue in life. I had dealt with the worst possible event that I could experience, and I was able to move forward. It made everything else seem easy in comparison. I try to remember that now as I move forward in life. I have experienced true loss so everything else can be conquered.

Although I had a new outlook and a better understanding of my own mortality I still had not formed an immediate need to get in shape. I was, after all, only 25 years old. I thought I can always get into shape later. I continued to lie to myself and tell myself that I would get into shape soon. I would start next week, and then things would change. I didn't see this as a problem because I was young and I had many years ahead of me. That, however, was the problem!

No matter what happened, I always had the excuse that I was young and could always do it later. Nothing kills your goals like procrastination. The sad thing is I may have continued to put off getting in shape and changing my life if I had not come to some simple realizations thanks to movies and a coworker.

5

Mullins, James Mullins

"How soon 'not now' becomes 'never.'"
– Martin Luther

How did a movie and a co-worker inspire me to become fit? Well, this was not the type of inspiration were someone sets a good example and became a mentor. This was a coworker who was the picture perfect example of what I was going to be if I didn't change.

My co-worker was about 10-15 years older than me, and he was about 125-150lbs overweight. He got around well and didn't have health problems so it wasn't the fact that he wasn't in great shape that changed my perspective. It wasn't pity or sympathy that woke me up. It was talking with him and hearing him always mention making changes and getting in shape. It was the constant false promises he was making to himself that made me realize I was making those same mistakes.

I promised myself that I would change just like he had promised himself that he would change for years. I could see myself doing the same thing. I could see myself buying equipment and not using it, lying to myself and saying I was going to change, making excuses and not living up to my commitments I made to myself. This continued until one night when I was watching a movie.

Have you ever seen someone else and wondered "Why can't I look like that?" Have you ever wanted to be like the movie stars? Have you ever looked at someone older and realized that they were in much better shape and healthier than you?

I have, I was watching Casino Royale starring Daniel Craig. There is a scene where he comes out of the ocean to meet with a woman he is going to try to seduce, and he is in phenomenal shape. Now I know, you must be thinking, why is this guy talking about Daniel Craig. Isn't this the type of thing that women should be talking about.

Well, it wasn't the physical attraction that caught my attention. It was his age. For some reason, something clicked inside my head that said: "He is in great shape for his age." Then I thought about it. How old is he?

Craig just happened to be around the same age as my co-worker/friend who kept talking to me about getting in shape. Here was a friend that I was communicating with daily and making routine false promises to get into shape. I began to think about my own appearance and all of our false promises.

Even though I was around 15 years younger than Daniel Craig, I was nowhere near his physique physically and not because I don't have the physical traits to compare but because I wasn't putting in the time or effort. I began to wonder, had my friend been making these promises since he was my age. Had he seen someone when he was younger that he looked at and said: "I can do that, I can get into shape like him."

I could clearly look at these two individuals and see that they had taken two different approaches to their physique and health. I then thought about my own path. Was I going to keep promising myself that I was going to get into shape without taking action? Was I going to end up like my friend? Or was I going to start taking action and attain the healthy and fit physique that I had envisioned?

I decided to choose the latter. My father passing had given me the perspective that change was needed. It had allowed me to begin to review things and understand that I couldn't continue to do the same things that I was in the past and expect different results.

This second realization with my co-worker had jarred me out of the stupor I was in and triggered the need to take action now. You see it is one thing to realize that change is needed. My experience with my dad had shown me that health was important, and I needed change. However, it is a totally different thing to realize that knowing you need to change is not enough.

You may know you need to change, but if you don't take action, it will be too late. I knew it was time for a change! I knew that if I waited until I was 40-45 years old before I woke up and took action that it would be considerably harder. I decided to make a change now and at that point, my fitness transformation was about to begin.

6

How P90X changed my life?

"You will never change your life until you change something you do daily." - Mike Murdock

Luckily I had seen those annoying P90X commercials that ran 800 times each day. The consistent infomercial that was always running every morning when I got up. I was becoming brainwashed by Beachbody to use their products and it was just what I needed.

I am an introvert, I'm shy, and I would rather be alone or with small groups of people I care about. I find it hard to get out and go to the gym and socialize with everyone there. I am quiet, and I like to hang out in the back of the room and keep to myself.

As I mentioned before, I also had a horrible work schedule and found it very hard to find time to go to the gym. I worked overnights frequently and had a rotating schedule that made it nearly impossible to workout.

That's where P90X worked for me. Those infomercials sold me on all of the things I needed. The ability to train at home, minimal equipment (I already had it), and a schedule that I could dictate. It was the perfect fit for me.

Finally, my DVD set arrived and then the fun began. There was a huge manual and the diet plan was intimidating. This was a well put together program, and it did not seem suited for a beginner.

I could not do all of the exercises, I couldn't make it through the workouts, and I couldn't follow the diet. There was one thing I could do, though, and that was KEEP PUSHING PLAY! Just like Tony Horton said on the DVD "Keep pushing play" and continue to come back the next day. I could do that.

What about you? Have you had struggles where you didn't think you could do something? How did you progress? In the end was overcoming the obstacle as hard as you imagined? Do you have something you are working toward now? Can you break it down in a simple way so that you can be successful?

I couldn't, however, follow the diet. It was very detailed and complicated for someone who was not ready for that big of a diet change. I looked through all of the information and tried to find ways to improve my diet. I was able to do that. I remember just trying to use lean cuisine and other "healthy" options. Since they were lower in calories than what I was eating before, they started to make a difference. I made slight changes little by little and slowly started to get my diet in line with the exercise. It wasn't until years later that I finally got my nutrition figured out and knew the proper way to eat healthily.

The exercises were hard, I remember having to hold my legs up on the leg scissors, but I kept doing them. The yoga was very long and plyometrics were very intense. There were exercises that I couldn't do at the end of the program and sometimes I would miss a workout, but I kept coming back.

Since I was struggling with some of the exercises and I wanted results, I started becoming more active with other types of training and cardio to help burn calories. I started practicing martial arts, running and playing some sports again. I kept at it, and I kept going and pushing toward my goal. The sad part is I wasn't educated enough actually to set a goal. I didn't have an end goal in mind. I didn't have a set number of pounds or inches to work toward. I just followed the plan. Record at 30 days, a record at 60 days record at 90 days.

I got great results! Looking back now, I know I should have set clear goals. I have a much better understanding of goal setting strategies and progress structure and having these set points to measure progress and being able to celebrate my accomplishments along the way would have helped my motivation. But I was a beginner and didn't understand these concepts. I just kept showing up and putting in the work.

I lost around 20lbs in my 90 days of P90X (with some added sports, cardio, and activity). It wasn't the weight loss and body transformation that I appreciate the most (I've lost more weight at later times once I got diet and exercise figured out). It was the mentality change, and the belief in myself that completing the program gave me that I valued the most.

By completing that program, it allowed me to see that if I stick to a goal, and I am focused I can see results. It made me start down a path to become better physically and mentally and to continue to grow and try to achieve the best body and mind possible for myself.

It increased my confidence and self-belief and if not for that program I would not have taken the steps necessary to forge my own path in fitness. I would not have done the research and put the hours of training in to become a coach, and I would not have developed the love for fitness that I have.

I am thankful for Tony Horton and his infomercials because at a time when I was looking for a way to make a change they were on the television. This small thing started me on a very important path.

I hope if you decide to make a similar change you allow me the pleasure and honor of helping you achieve your goals!

Due to the importance of P90X to my life, I wanted to share this story with you. I also wanted to include a similar program with some of the same principles so you can try them out and see if circuit training programs are suited for you.

7

Beginning to Run

"Believe that you can run farther or faster. Believe that you're young enough, old enough, strong enough, and so on to accomplish everything you want to do. Don't let worn-out beliefs stop you from moving beyond yourself." — John Bingham

When I decided that I wanted to get in better shape and lose weight, I knew that burning more calories was going to be the way to do that. I didn't know what calorie deficits were or the reason to be in a calorie deficit but I knew exercise and activity were important.

While P90X was a starting point, I also began to run to try to be more active and increase my daily calorie burn. I wanted to do P90X and run in conjunction to use running as an extra aid in the fat loss.

Have you ever tried running for exercise? Have you tried outdoor activities? Have you ever participated in a race? Do you think you may enjoy meeting others who help and support one another?

My wife and I live near a local park which allows me to have access to fields, trails, and sidewalks to run on. Having played basketball, I knew how beneficial running was to conditioning so I thought I would start. I was very unaware of what the fitness aspect of running involved.

While running plays a major role in sports it is not necessarily a focus for the coaching staff. Since we were a small school and did not have a strength and conditioning coach our running was not structured or analyzed in any way. I was involved in sports before performance improvement became the norm. Our coaches didn't have the resources and education that is available today for planning a structured endurance program.

There was no one to educate me on the proper form of running or how to prevent injury. All of our running was done at high intensity. The programs were not structured with progression and rest and often we were not allowed water except at certain points in practice. While this may seem strange now, it was the standard practice at the time because the science and performance had not been communicated to the coaches. No one had shown how better hydration, progression, and recovery could improve the teams of that era.

This left me at a disadvantage when I decided to begin running to get into better shape as an adult. I had this crazy thought that I could just take off running, and it would be easy. After all, we are designed to run as a species.

I can tell you from experience if you are overweight and out of shape you are not just "ready to run!" Not only was I an inexperienced runner but I decided to get an extra calorie burn during my first run by wearing a 20lb weighted vest.

So, I take off from my house and begin my jog to the park. By the time I arrive on the first hill I realize just how out of shape I actually am. I'm stubborn, which at times can be a good thing, so even though I couldn't run the whole trail I walked it and finished my goal distance for the day.

Once I finished and arrived home, I was exhausted. The next day I almost couldn't move. This was the wake up that I needed. It not only taught me to take my time with running and allow for steady progress but it also taught me the same lessons for P90X. This lesson of easing into new things and making sure you allow yourself to grow and learn is something I have adopted in every other fitness and self-improvement goal I set moving forward.

This is where I learned that not being able to do the initial thing that I set out to do was not a failure. Failure would have been quitting! It would have been stopping when it got hard. I not only finished by walking the distance I set out, but I learned from my experience that the weighted vest was too much and that I was in worse shape than I thought.

Moving forward I knew that I needed to progress slowly. I understood that slow progress was progress and that as long as I was moving forward, I wasn't standing still. I still didn't know how to progress my running program, but I knew that I couldn't go about things the way I began. This led to my investigation on how to improve at running.

Now you have to understand that I hated running. I just knew it would help get me in shape. I knew that it would help me lose body fat quicker. So I looked for ways to get better. I continued to run with the only intent being to stay in shape and improve my cardiovascular health.

Then once again, a co-worker made a difference. He started chatting with me about running. He said he wanted to start and that he wanted to run in a 5k race. Now as I said before, I'm not much of a fan of being in crowds or being around strangers. So, I was hesitant but I like to encourage anyone to improve and become involved with fitness, so I agreed that if he signed up, I would join him.

This is how my yearly participation in the Charleston Distance Run began. If you ever get a chance, you should come and participate. I only participate in the 5k since running isn't my primary fitness goal. There are several races including a 15-mile race for experienced runners. My friend, Mike, didn't end up being able to compete that first year because of injury (he has since completed the 15-mile race), but because I had already paid for my participation, I decided to proceed.

I am glad that I did. It allowed me to overcome some of the fear of the involvement in a public event, and it allowed me to develop a way that I could compete against myself while running. After I saw my initial finishing time each year I made a personal goal to beat my previous year.

This led to increased research on running and programming and different ways to improve my performance. I started tracking various aspects and utilizing tools to improve. Through this experience, I gained valuable knowledge to help when it came time for my strength and conditioning certification.

Not only did race participation help with my running education but it allowed me to see how others treated each other in the running community and saw the atmosphere around events. I witnessed how supportive the runners were for the other racers. Seeing the many people participating and helping each other is very moving. I also enjoy hearing about the participants and finding out their different reasons for participation. Hearing these stories is very inspirational.

There are many inspiring people and stories at running events that I would suggest any time you can be involved in a race that you chose to support the event. You will enjoy it!

Since I like the atmosphere and now know others that are participating, I continue to run in this race each year. After I gained more knowledge about running, I understand how to structure programs, and it is not as miserable an experience as I once thought. I run now mainly as a way to relax because I enjoy being outside and I can't resistance train through the park.

To ensure you don't go through the same struggles that I did and take off in a weighted vest, I have included some walking and running programs to get you on your way. They are constructed with gradual progression and ensure the growing process is easier than mine.

I hope you use them and that you develop an enjoyment for running. It is a relaxing, cheap, and enjoyable way to get outdoors and enjoy life. But only, if you do it right!

8

The Next Karate ~~Kid~~ Adult

"If you always put limit on everything you do, physical or anything else. It will spread into your work and into your life. There are no limits. There are only plateaus, and you must not stay there, you must go beyond them."

- Bruce Lee

After my time developing a steady running program I decided to look for other ways to get cardiovascular exercise and burn extra fat. I never was a die-hard runner, and I have always looked for other ways to burn calories. Sports allowed me to do that when I was younger but, now that I have grown older, it is harder to find people willing to participate.

In a pursuit for solo sporting options, I was led to martial arts. Like many men my age I loved Chuck Norris when I was younger. I also I had an uncle who studied and participated in Karate. My uncle (whom I am named after) died at a young age and my mother always talked about his love for martial arts. We also had pictures of him in his Gi up at our home and seeing him in his uniform always made me wonder what the sport was like. These influences always made me interested in pursuing martial arts. Growing up in our small community meant that martial arts were not readily available, and it was not an option for me during my youth.

As an adult I was looking for any way to be active and I had the chance to begin Karate. I joined USA Martial Arts and began my training.

They offered many different styles, and I could attend many different classes several days a week. They also offered some basic self-defense techniques at the classes in addition to the traditional martial arts styles. I really enjoyed the classes and the physicality but being an introvert, it was always a struggle to force myself to go to class. I always enjoyed participating, and I was always glad that I went but getting motivated to go was a struggle.

Do you have limits that you set for yourself? What major fears do you have? Why do they bother you? What can you do to move past them? If you overcome them how will that help you reach your goals?

Socializing and crowds have always been a struggle for me but let this be a lesson on overcoming fear or discomfort and allowing yourself to grow. I had to get used to being uncomfortable and around others to participate in something I enjoyed. This has happened to me frequently in life. There have even been times in certain situations where I actually drive to the location and will not go in to participate.

Now, when this occurs you might get the mental picture of me being worried or nervous and wanting to avoid the situation. Being nervous isn't exactly how I would describe it. What would happen is I would drive to the venue, find a place to park, and get ready to enter. Since I always try to arrive at all of my appointments early, I always have time to sit in the car for a few minutes and think. This moment while I sit in my car and prepare to enter the event I would go through a thought process that I think most people experience and I want to share it with you so that if you have similar problems it might help you relate to someone else and overcome this obstacle.

I would sit there and begin to make reasons in my mind of why I shouldn't attend the class. Like I said this has happened to me on several occasions. I begin to make excuses. I think things like: "What are we going to do today?" "Should I be at home doing _____ instead?" "I attended class Monday I can skip today" "You are tired why don't you just rest and recuperate?"

You see, all of these thoughts, all of these mental barriers, I was putting in front of myself are excuses. These are really defense mechanisms that I am making to avoid the discomfort I have from social situations. It is fear keeping me from growing and allowing me to stay in my comfort zone of my home and near familiar people who I trust.

This isn't how you grow; this isn't how you become better. Fear and limiting beliefs are a major problem that everyone will face. If you are starting to realize that you may be building you own barriers or limiting yourself, don't feel alone. As you can see everyone does it.

Those limits don't have to be like mine. They don't have to be about crowds or social situations. You can look at the questions and reasons I was giving myself for not going to class to participate, and you can see how that can relate to other situations.

How many times has someone wanted to start an exercise program, take an educational class, or apply for a promotion and let limiting beliefs, fear, and negativity get in the way? How many times have you asked yourself similar questions like "Do I deserve this?" Am I good enough to accomplish this?" What if I fail?"

Please understand everyone has similar thoughts at some point. Those who achieve success find ways to overcome these thoughts. Your thoughts are not who you are, and they are not you actions. They are merely ideas in your head, and you have total control over how to use them.

You see people think that the thoughts they have defined them, but it is their actions that define us. This is what courage is. Everyone has fear. Courage is having the thought and emotional response of fear then realizing you feel it, understanding it, and taking action against it.

The only difference in the courageous and the cowardly is the actions taken. Not the presence of fear. So if you find yourself struggling to take an action understand this and take action to move forward.

The issue I faced as in introvert in social situations has nothing to do with fear of the people involved. Almost everyone in fitness, public speaking, or in your career are usually very supportive.

A great piece of advice I received about public speaking that relates to many other situations is this: "The audience doesn't want you to fail. They are rooting for you to succeed." Think about that. In most situations, if you take the perspective of the other person, they do want you to succeed. They are putting time and effort into being there, and they like to share in your success so why would they want you to fail.

This sentiment also applies to other areas in life. Life is not a zero-sum game, and more than one person can be successful. This allows many people to be positive and supportive of you and your goals. So it wasn't about the people. It was just about the effort and energy that I have to put out to go outside of my comfort zone.

This is definitely something an extrovert would not understand, but it is something I would go through frequently. The mental dread of being around a group of people even when there is no judgment or negativity is still energy draining for an introvert.

Even today, to continue to grow, I still try to overcome this hurdle. Being an introvert is something I continue to deal with, but it is easier now than it used to be. Participating in martial arts not only allowed me to be active but also work on this aspect of my personality.

Anyway, back to how karate relates to my fitness journey. I continued to take Karate for around a year, but I began to have schedule problems that interfered. Not only was getting to classes becoming a problem but USA Martial Arts also requires their participants to participate in two tournaments each year. I was only trying to learn and gain experience, and since I was near 30 years old, I was not interested in tournament participation. My work schedule also required overnights which coincided with the tournament schedule. Without the time to prepare for the tournaments, I could not meet the needed yearly requirements to progress. After reviewing my options, I decided to pursue other forms of activity.

9

Self-Defense & Self Development

"To fight and conquer in all our battles is not supreme excellence; supreme excellence consists in breaking the enemy's resistance without fighting."

- Sun Tzu

After participating in CrossFit for a few years (Don't worry, I'll discuss Crossfit eventually) and learning different ways to minimize my time in the gym I decided to look once again into Martial Arts. I wanted to get a black belt and still planned to pursue it at some point. Since I felt too old to compete in a Karate tournament, I looked for other areas of Martial Arts for my cardiovascular activity. After looking into several styles, I decided on Krav Maga. Krav Maga gives you a great workout with constant movement, and it is designed to be completely about self-defense. Since I am an adult, I feel that learning a sport for competition at this point in my life is not beneficial. I also find many benefits in someone being capable of defending oneself so Krav Maga made an excellent choice.

After some research, I decided to choose Premier Martial Arts. After meeting Brian Lucas, the owner and head instructor, I knew that I had selected to perfect place for me to learn and grow. Brian has years of experience in many different styles of Martial Arts and is also an expert in Gun Training, Wildlife Training, and Survival. He is pretty much a one-man survival machine, and I enjoy being around him. He is an excellent teacher and really helped me grow as a student and as a person.

Krav Maga added a great cardio component to my normal resistance training, and I was in the best shape of my life. Krav Maga in addition to my normal strength program was an excellent way to stay well-conditioned and remain strong. Krav Maga is great exercise and improves both your power and conditioning.

I took Krav Maga for over a year, and I really enjoyed learning the movements and defenses. I also enjoyed fending off multiple attackers and weapon defenses. Participating in Krav Maga will definitely prepare you to defend yourself if you are ever in a bad situation.

I have included some basic Krav Maga with the Karate portion in the Martial Arts Training Workout to allow you to experience some of the benefits of Krav Maga. It really requires a combatant or attacker to understand the complete benefits. You will not get the same workout or experience without a partner. I wanted to include at least a few items for you to try and allow you to experience a portion of each of the major aspects of fitness that I have utilized along my fitness journey. You never know which one you may fall in love with that becomes the life changing activity you have been looking for.

While taking Krav Maga, I also started taking some pistol defense classes from Brian and with the relationship we formed I began to learn more about him and his entrepreneur background. I had already begun studying for my Strength and Conditioning Certification as a hobby, and I was thinking of ways to use it professionally. I had also started listening to a podcast called Barbell Business about owning and running a gym.

I knew I had the fitness knowledge and capabilities to be a trainer and coach and with my business management background, I felt that I had many of the qualities needed to run a successful business. While participating in the self-defense classes and talking to Brian, I was also gaining the confidence needed to begin my own business journey.

Brian was sharing his personal business experiences with me and giving me input to help me develop in both business and martial arts. He also had a similar career path to the one I was aspiring to take. He became not only a martial arts instructor but also a mentor that could help me with my other goals in life. After much research and talking with Brian, I decided I may want to start my own business.

10

What is CrossFit?

"Intelligence is the ability to adapt to change." -
Stephen Hawking

After deciding to step away from Karate, but before my involvement in Krav Maga, I was still looking for ways to stay active. I am always looking for more information and resources about training and this curiosity and love for learning led me to CrossFit. I started to get involved with CrossFit early in its existence, and I thought it was great.

I was already using many different modes of training that were being used in CrossFit like Plyometrics and Circuit Training. I had not gotten deeply involved with Olympic Lifting or Gymnastics, so this was a nice change of pace.

Living in a small city limited the available options available for Crossfit. Crossfit was just growing at that point, and there were no Crossfit gyms in our area. Had I been more confident and better educated in the business aspects of fitness and entrepreneurship I may have been able to see this wave of popularity coming and been able to get on board.

Unfortunately, I missed the boat with the business aspect but at least I found the fitness part early and found ways to utilize it for my own personal growth. Even though there were not any affiliates nearby I had many of the tools and resources available to begin utilizing some of the Crossfit programs.

CrossFit posts daily workouts on its website and as a workout junkie, it was a great way for me to get more programs. I started trying to add these in with my other programs. If I was performing a bodybuilding program I would try to incorporate CrossFit into off days. If I was strapped for time, I would just do the Workout of the Day.

I soon realized that I was not as "fit" as I thought. I could run and I could lift considerable weight, but I wasn't well rounded. CrossFit made me want to be. It also came into my life at a great time because it gave me a way to get in quicker workouts when I wanted to, and that was important. I was tired of spending hours at the gym and then running for the cardiovascular benefits.

Being involved in CrossFit also made me want to learn more about the movement and mobility portions of exercise. I had always enjoyed the science of exercise, but I had never looked at the movement or mobility the way I had to to understand the Gymnastics and Olympic movements.

CrossFit also had some great coaching through the online site which made me want to find out more about all aspects of fitness. This was the first time coaching was really made available to a mass audience, and it allowed us all to grow because of it. If you have never been to a CrossFit class (we have since had several affiliates open in my area), you should defiantly go and try it. It is an excellent program and great for extroverts.

However, as an introvert, I was not well suited for the classes. I preferred to train at home and utilize the workouts from the website. I also began to look at some other programs from other strength coaches and other websites. I started using programs from T-Nation, Mark Rippetoe, Jim Wendler, and others.

I really enjoyed CrossFit and I still use metabolic conditioning in my training, but I have moved away from the gymnastics portions. CrossFit does not lend itself to home training very well. You can't always find a rope to climb or gymnastic rings at home. I find it hard to make time to travel to the gym and participate, and it is much more convenient for me to train at home. So I only utilize training that I can do at home which means much of the gymnastics portion is out of the question.

I was able to continue to utilize the Olympic lifts and find ways to strength train at home. I loved the strength training programs that I discovered and used them with metabolic conditioning was becoming my preference. I tried to find ways to incorporate strength training into circuit training on a regular basis. This love for learning and growth and the need for quicker more intense workouts led to CrossFit, which helped led me to Strength and Conditioning.

11

Transforming My Self & My Life

"When I let go of what I am, I become what I might be." - Lao Tzu

I look at my complete transformation as a three-part journey. At my heaviest, I was 250lbs and me slowly over an unmeasured period of time lost 20-25lbs. I saw amazing results from my transformation. Over a six-month span, I lost 40-45lbs. This averages to about 7lbs per month. Now I would like to attribute my transformation to some great six-month program but I can't. I didn't follow a specific program throughout, and it was not over a continuous sixth month period.

My initial 20lb weight loss was a three-month process that involved P90X with running and other activities mixed in. I spend a lot of time after that learning about fitness and developing my own programs. I was around 205lbs, and I was happy with the weight I lost so I didn't cut any more weight.

While continuing to exercise and participate in various other activities like the ones I have discussed earlier I began to dig deeper into the educational aspects of fitness. I found university programs on ITunesU and textbooks and began to study in depth. I was not satisfied with my years of studying videos, magazine, books, podcasts, and gym participation. I wanted to know the how the science of exercise applied to what I had already learned, and I wasn't happy with the information I had gathered up until this point.

After I had learned enough and tried many other programs, I decided to see how I could progress with my own three-month program. I structured it around the strength and conditioning principles I had learned. I utilized strength training, metabolic conditioning, and undulated training to form a program that I thought should give solid results. I also focused in on my nutrition and made sure it was in perfect order so that I would get the best results. This is how I lost the remainder of the weight and finally got to my leanest 180lbs.

This equated to a 25lb weight loss over a three-month span. So with the results from this portion and the P90X portion, I managed to lose 40-45lbs over a six-month span. This isn't exceptional weight loss. Most people should be able to achieve similar results. It averages out to less than 2lbs per week, and that is a realistic, healthy, and achievable goal.

Now, most people would think that at 6'1" and 180lbs is too thin. I tend to agree as I prefer to be closer to 200lbs, but I was still muscular and didn't lose much strength. I think I look skinny at 180lbs, and I like a little more size so I stay around 200lbs even though it means I carry a little more body fat. I figure as long as I can see some visible abs I am good with my body fat percentage. Whenever they start to fade, I readjust my diet to get my body fat back in line.

With the strength and conditioning program, I developed I managed to have the following stats. All of this, mind you, is at the lowest weight and most lean that I have been.

Height 6'1."	Weight 180lbs	Waist 35."
Hips 34."	Neck 17."	Biceps 16.25."
Forearm 13."	Calf 14."	Thigh 23."
Chest 44." 10%	Shoulders 55."	BF Estimate-8-

Deadlift-435lbs   Squat-405lbs   Bench-285lbs

5k time-23:55

Trust me, I'm not posting stats because I think they are something special. There are many people who have a much better body and can lift much more weight. I prefer not to discuss numbers and would rather discuss the benefits from results such as the ability to carry more groceries or play sports without being winded.

The reason I wanted to share some of my results is so that you can see that a regular Joe, who was working swing shifts and working out at home, can build a decent physique with respectable strength stats. You can do something similar and like me, you can do it at home and around your schedule.

Developing my own routine and seeing good results led me to believe that I could do the same for others. This was when I decided to get certified and become a coach.

After self-education with videos and textbooks, I finally felt like I was ready to join a program for certification. This was yet another education process, but it was one I was well prepared for.

After looking for the most valued and highly accredited exercise certification organizations, I decided upon the National Strength & Conditioning Association. I had previously studied the NSCA Certified Personal Trainer material but I wanted to learn more about strength training, so I decided to become a Certified Strength & Conditioning Specialist. Luckily, I had prepared well, and their program included many things that I had already learned on my own. This put me in a very comfortable mindset for the certification exam.

After finishing the course, I went to take my exam so I could take the steps to become a coach and start trying to form a business. I performed very well on my exam and passed without problems becoming a Certified Strength & Conditioning Coach.

At this point, I felt ready and started to coach some friends and put together a business plan to open my own gym.

Once again, I turned to ItunesU, podcasts, and books for my education. I value learning but unfortunately things are set up to make education either unattainable or leaving you indebted to lenders. While the education you receive in college is worthwhile, there is also a wealth of free information available now. As I mentioned before Barbell Business was an excellent help with my understanding of business and the confidence and the lectures and programs on ItunesU helped with education.

I continued to study and develop and seek more information about the financial and advertising parts of my current management position. I also joined the local Small Business Development Center and went to meet with a business coach to help with forming a game plan for my business. Everyone there was very helpful and also warned of the hardships that starting a business entailed. I am very thankful to have had this help as it really prepared me for the process of moving forward.

After much research and development, I had a plan and was ready to present to the bank. The day of my meeting, things didn't go as planned. I am always early for everything but wouldn't you know that I had problems getting the final plan from the company I was working with, getting it printed, and being ready to present.

I ended up being 10 minutes late for my meeting. I know this looked bad and was a poor impression, but I had to have the items I printed, and I didn't expect the printing problems. I had allowed plenty of time, but the problems had overtaken even the extra time I had allotted.

Have you ever run into multiple obstacles that you didn't think you could overcome? Have you ever felt like nothing would go right and that you have no control over the outcome? Have you ever felt like just giving up?

I expected things to go poorly, but they didn't. I had a great meeting, and things went well. The banker told me I was one of the most prepared people he had worked with and that the plan was excellent.

He also happened to be from a small town near where I grew up so we chatted and had things in common allowing us to form a connection. I was very pleased, and confident things would turn out well.

It didn't. The underwriters wouldn't approve the loan because they didn't want me to leave my job to run a gym. They didn't think I would have adequate cash flow to pay them and myself even though I had asked for enough working capital to cover all of the costs I needed.

I was hugely disappointed. I knew I could help others, I knew the plan was solid, and I knew I could run this business well. I also knew my local area needed more people who were involved in fitness. I had a goal to be a coach and find a way to share my journey and help others get the same feeling and results that I did.

Have you ever had a major project or a really important goal that turned out badly? Have you ever worked very hard for success and failed? How did you handle that situation? Did you quit or did you use it to learn, grow, and move forward again?

So, not to be deterred I asked the bank how much I could get for a personal loan instead of a business loan. Now, this may seem like a bad idea, but I had such a belief in what I wanted to do and in trying to have an impact on others that I had to try.

I was involved in retail so long, and I had seen many people come in and buy items they didn't need. I worked in a toy store so I would see people come in and spend hundreds and thousands of dollars on toys. Things that weren't necessity.

To make things worse, I felt like I was adding to their problems by encouraging our team to sell them credit cards. Not only were they buying items they didn't need, but we were asking them to buy the stuff with money they didn't have.

Now I understand that this is a decision they make, and they want these items to solve a problem and need they have which is their child's happiness. It's just that I have a hard time feeling like I am having a positive impact on the world in that scenario.

Are you happy with your current situation in life? Do you feel like you are maximizing your potential? Are you happy with your health and your career? Do you have a burning desire to do more?

With this need to have an impact and make a difference in the world, I was willing to take a chance and get the personal loan. I still felt like I could make a difference.

The personal loan was not nearly enough for me to stick with my original plan so I had to restructure and go with an online business model with less overhead and expense. So that is what I did. I hired a business coach to help me develop this model and began to find ways to reach out to find people looking for help.

My business coach (his name is AJ Mihrzad at Online Super Coach if you want to check him out) and I worked together and started marketing. Finally, with his help, I began to get leads. I began to take calls and try to help people but had little luck getting clients. I am not a salesman. I have never been. I am a shy introvert, and I don't like to brag about myself, my programs, or my abilities (Yeah I know, I am writing a book, seems kinda braggy right?). So I struggled to get my first clients.

That's the hardest part as a new coach. Even though I had the abilities and wasn't out to take money from people without earning it, it's still hard to gain trust. You can have the desire and willingness to help others but people need convincing to believe in you. There are so many people who are trying to take advantage and misinforming people that when someone is honestly trying to help they have a hard time.

Well, I kept plugging away and I eventually I broke through. I started getting more leads and feeling more confident in everything I was doing. I decided to step away from the retail management job and take a chance on coaching.

I was stepping away from a job I had worked at since I was 21 years old. I had spent over 12 years there. It was my family and I loved the people there. I was sad about leaving and scared about starting a business. It was the hardest decision I have ever made.

The only thing that helped was I believed in my goal and knowing I could help others. I had confidence in myself. Because of fitness, I knew about goal setting, determination, and desire. I knew my goal, I knew that I could help make a difference and I had the desire to succeed so I made the leap and it changed my life.

Now there is a huge difference in what I was planning and what I ended up doing. I wanted to work in a group coaching setting and be in a gym all day. I ended up having to work one on one and in an office all day.

The important thing though is that the mission didn't change. My goal was to provide a positive, supportive, environment where people could feel comfortable working toward their fitness goals, and I do that on a daily basis.

There are many benefits for me with the online coaching model with only one drawback. I hate being in an office all day. I do like the freedom it allows me to have and the flexibility. I can work meetings and speak engagements around my schedule, and I can do my coaching from anywhere. I am not tied to a gym like I would have been otherwise.

Online coaching also offers more benefit to the people I help. Instead of a class based group learning session, there is more one on one coaching which allows more individual coaching access. I planned on opening a Crossfit affiliate which would have meant that clients only had their hour class to get their coaching and ask questions. The class format doesn't leave much time to discuss the mindset and nutritional strategies that are needed in addition to the training program.

The online coaching model gives the people coaching access to ask these questions and learn at their own pace. Coaching also offers a more flexible schedule, and they can work out at home.

These are all huge benefits for most people. Most people would prefer this business model to the one I was going to offer initially. The main thing is that it still allows me to help people get the results they want.

As you can see, there were many different obstacles and setbacks along the way. There were many times I could have quit and many times I wanted to. It was hard, and I felt like a failure many times. My wife was worried, and we had some financial issues, but I kept sticking to the plan. I knew what my goal was, I knew I could do it, I knew that I could help others live happier, healthier, and better lives. That is why I do it!

How does this relate to you and getting in shape? Well, I wanted you to see how the struggles and obstacles you run into during your fitness journey translate to the rest of your life. You can see many parallels between my fitness journey and my business journey. I want you to see that with the right mindset and planning that you too can take action and begin your journey. Not just a fitness journey but any journey you choose.

Semper Liberi means "always free" and I want to do everything I can to promote a freedom lifestyle not only with fitness but every area of life. If you are unfulfilled in any aspect of your life, and you want more, I want you to be inspired to take action to free yourself of any burdens holding you back.

This book is mainly about my fitness journey and programs to help you begin your own, but I also have included resources for you to dig deeper into entrepreneurship. I want you to have the starting point if you decide you want to follow a path similar to mine. I want you to believe that you can do unbelievable things. I want fitness just to be the starting point for all of the great things you achieve.

I want you to be inspired. I want you to get your health and fitness in order so you will be ready to tackle every other aspect of life. I want you to have more energy and be more capable of taking on any challenge. I want you to become mentally, physically, and emotionally stronger.

I hope you have found many things through this book that inspire you. I hope you look at a shy, introvert, from a small town who most people would assume couldn't be a successful coach and speaker and see how you can do it too.

I hope you look at the chubby kid turned overweight college kid that had a life changing event and relate somehow. I hope you see his transformation and think you can do it too.

I hope you see the inexperienced retail worker who made a leap of faith and started his own business and thought you can do it too.

I hope you see my fitness journey and think you can do it too.

I know you can! I did it, you can too!

Part 2 – How to utilize the programs.

The goal of the programs I have included in this book is to give you a way to start your fitness journey. I don't believe in a one size fits all approach to health and fitness. I think that programs vary as much as the individual participating in them.

Everyone has different things they enjoy and different movement patterns. This means that every program might not be suitable for every individual. With this in mind, I wanted to give you samples of programs so you could try them and choose what type of training you enjoy.

Think of this as a sampler platter and your beginning one of these training styles full time as the main course. These programs are all designed as a beginner program with a one-week sample included.

This sample program can be repeated, and you will continue to see results, but they are not set up to be long term programs. Long term programs are designed with progression in mind and have peaks and valleys of training levels to allow you to adapt, recover, and progress.

If you decide to utilize these programs long term, make sure you incorporate a deload(rest) week once a month. At some point, you will progress past these programs and need to seek other ways to progress.

There are many other types of fitness programs and sports available to help get, and keep, you in shape. Because I have tried so many different methods and have so many interests I wanted to share the programs I am the most familiar with, in hopes that you will find something you enjoy and cut out the need for you searching on your own. However, if there isn't an activity here that you enjoy don't be deterred. There are so many fitness options available, and you will definitely be able to find something that you enjoy.

My goal was to share my fitness experiences and give you a way to see some of the many things fitness has to offer. I have never seen a collection of programs similar to this, and I thought it would be helpful to those looking for a program to suit their needs. This should allow a nice variety of selection and make it easier for you to find something you enjoy.

Please use these as a way to see what types of training are available, find one you enjoy, and then move into participating into it with the proper coaching and guidance. The goal of this book is to get you to take action and move forward toward your goal. I have included enough variety so that you should find a training program that you enjoy. You have to take action and start the journey.

I want you to have all of the beginning steps so that you can start a path to health and fitness as well as developing your career and personal development. My journey should have given you some insight into the many ways I have grown and developed through my experiences.

While I cannot give you step-by-step instructions here for business or personal success, I do want to ensure that you have some of the resources that I have used for my own personal development.

With these resources, you will have a head start that I didn't have, and it will save you a significant portion of time and effort if you decide to pursue an entrepreneurial career.

Here are some great resources to pursue both the fitness programs and entrepreneurship further.

Websites

P90X – A link for P90X.

www.crossfit.com – Find an affiliate near you.

www.mobilitywod.com - The best place for mobility guidance.

www.myfitnesspal.com - My favorite food tracking app.

www.argus.com – A great activity tracker.

www.slf.fit – Use our program selector tool and find the best type of fitness program for you.

www.slf.fit/free - Our free program page. You can get more exercise programs there.

www.slf.fit/join - Our membership sign-up page.

www.premiermartialarts.com – Find a martial arts dojo near you.

www.nsca.com – If you want to look into being a strength coach or personal trainer.

Just in case you are interested in beginning a business here are a few links to get you started.

https://www.liveplan.com – Get your business plan.

www.legalzoom.com – To form your business and get legal resources

www.irs.gov – Visit them and set up tax info. Also, visit your state tax site and set up the needed forms.

www.onlinesupercoach.com – My 1st online coach.

www.internetbusinessmastery.com – An excellent internet business resource.

www.SBDC.com – You want to find your local area Small Business Development Center

www.PTDC.com – Personal Trainer Development Center -Another great fitness training resource.

www.slmanage.com – The Sales & Leadership for Management learning resource I developed to help others succeed in management.

www.scribd.com – A great monthly book program where you can gain access to audio books and digital books for a monthly fee.

www.audible.com – Another great audiobook application.

www.amazon.com – Check out Kindle Unlimited to get the best value in digital books.

Books

Fitness & Training

Starting Strength – Mark Rippetoe and Jason Kelly – The place to start when learning strength training.

Practical Programming – Mark Rippetoe and Andy Baker – A great resource for learning to program for strength training.

Becoming A Supple Leopard – Kelly Starrett - Excellent modality guide.

Ready To Run – Kelly Starrett – A guide to getting you ready and keep you healthy during running.

5/3/1 – Jim Wendler - My favorite strength training program.

The New Encyclopedia of Modern Bodybuilding – Arnold Schwarzenegger – A must have if you want to learn about building a great physique.

Business

The 4-Hour Work Week – Timothy Ferris – **The book that made me think** I could have a business.

Rich Dad Poor Dad – Robert Kiyosaki – **A book everyone should read** to learn about money and how it is perceived.

Think and Grow Rich – Napoleon Hill – **A guide to success that has** principles you can use in every facet of life.

How to Win Friends & Influence People – Daniel Carnegie – **A great** resource to help you understand people and how to interact and communicate in constructive ways. It is useful for anyone who needs to communicate efficiently in business or in life.

The 7 Habits of Highly Effective People – Stephen R. Covey – **More** principles to help you succeed. I use them in planning both my business goals and fitness goals.

The One Thing – Gary Keller & Jay Papasan – **A great book that will** help you focus on the most important things that you need to do to ensure success.

These are just a few of the many resources that I have used along the way, but it is enough to get you started and well on your journey toward success. If you want more great book recommendations, you can check out my list on Goodreads.

Part 3 – The programs

Warm-Up

First, I am going to start off with the Warm-up program. This is just a sample warm-up that can be utilized before any of these programs to get you loose and ready to train.

Always make sure to warm-up before beginning any fitness program to help improve safety and performance. You also want to consult with your doctor before beginning any training program or diet plan and ensure that it will be safe for you and your health needs.

Use this program and warm-up for at least 5-minutes. After warming up, you can begin to work on mobility before training. Take 10 minutes and address any mobility issues or tight muscle you have. After performing your mobility work, you should then be ready to choose a program and begin your workout.

Cool Down

For the cool down portion of any workout, you can utilize the warm-up again as a means to wind down, or you can use some of the exercises from Circuit Program 2 – Program 2 which is designed to develop mobility and flexibility.

This program is a complete workout, but you can take a few exercises and use them as a cool down for whatever workout you complete. Make sure to choose exercises that focus on the muscles you worked during your workout or any muscles that may have flexibility or mobility problems. Addressing this area during the cool down period is an excellent way to reduce soreness and also improve mobility.

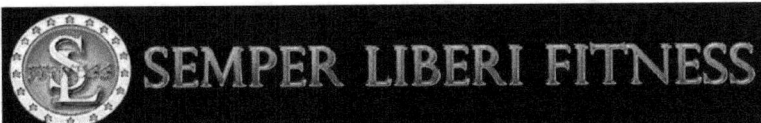

Phase: Warm-up - Program 1

A1 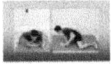 **Dynamic 90/90 Glute Stretch**
Sets: 1 Reps: 30sec

A2 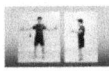 **Swinging Pectoral Stretch**
Sets: 1 Reps: 30sec

A3 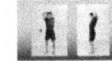 **Dynamic Triceps Overhead Stretch**
Sets: 1 Reps: 30sec

A4 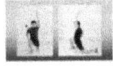 **Lunging Hip Flexor Stretch**
Sets: 1 Reps: 30sec

A5 **Swinging Hamstring Stretch**
Sets: 1 Reps: 30sec

A6 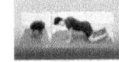 **Moving Cat Stretch**
Sets: 1 Reps: 30sec

A7 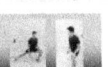 **Dynamic Adductor Stretch**
Sets: 1 Reps: 30sec

A8 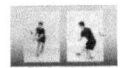 **Dynamic Biceps Femoris Stretch**
Sets: 1 Reps: 30sec

A9 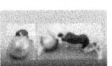 **Dynamic Lat Stretch on Swiss Ball**
Sets: 1 Reps: 30sec

A10  **Dynamic Pectoral Stretch**
Sets: 1 Reps: 30sec

A11 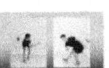 **Dynamic Semimembranosus Stretch**
Sets: 1 Reps: 30sec

Phase: Warm-up - Program 1

A1 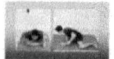 **Dynamic 90/90 Glute Stretch**
Sets: 1 Reps: 30sec

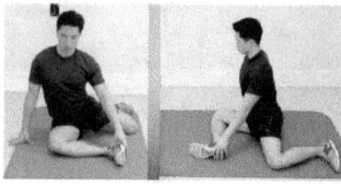 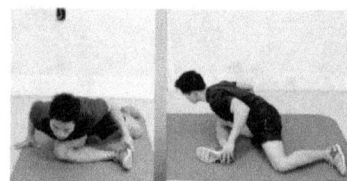

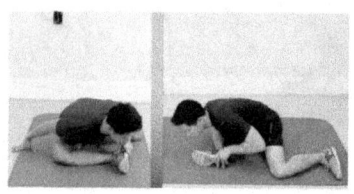

- Sit with one leg out in front of your hips and one leg behind. Bend both knees to 90 degrees.

- Lean forward to just outside your front knee.

- Use your outside arm to push your torso in towards your front foot. You should feel a stretch in the bum, lower back and outside of your front leg as you move your body across your leg.

- Lift your torso up to release the stretch and repeat the movement.

A2 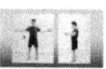 **Swinging Pectoral Stretch**
Sets: 1 Reps: 30sec

61

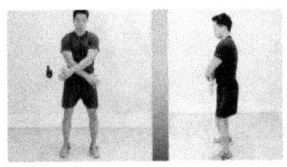 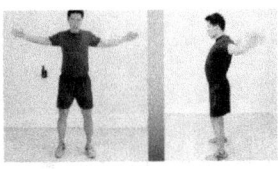

- Stand with your arms out in front of your shoulders and palms facing each other.

- Swing your arms out to the sides and back behind your shoulders to get a stretch in your chest.

- Swing your arms in front of your body before coming back out again.

- Push the stretch a little further with each repetition.

A3 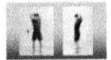 **Dynamic Triceps Overhead Stretch**
Sets: 1 Reps: 30sec

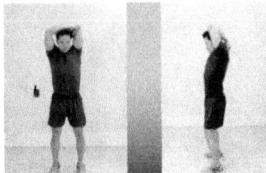 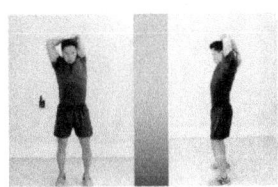

- Stand with feet hip width apart. Lift one arm overhead and bend at the elbow to bring the palm of your hand down behind your neck. Keep your elbow up above your shoulder.

- Use your other hand to apply pressure to the elbow pulling it in and down. You should feel a stretch at the back of your arm.

- Hold for a second and then release the stretch.

- Increase the stretch with each repetition.

A4 **Lunging Hip Flexor Stretch**

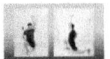 Sets: 1 Reps: 30sec

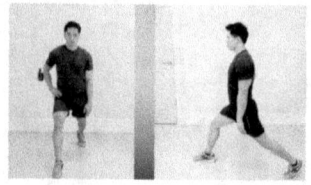 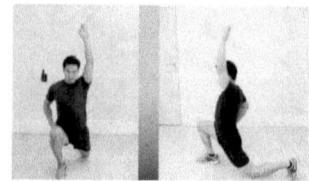

- Push your chest up and draw in your tummy with 30% effort. Step forward approximately 1 ½ times your normal stride length.

- Putting your weight on your front leg, lower yourself forward and down.

- As you come down, push your hips forward, squeeze your bum and raise the arm corresponding with your back leg straight above your shoulder. You should feel a good stretch in front of your hip on the back leg

- Keep your head and chest upright with your hips level and forward facing during the whole movement.

- Repeat the movement on the same leg gradually increasing the stretch.

- Once complete one the first leg repeat the process on the other.

A5 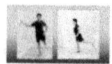 **Swinging Hamstring Stretch**
Sets: 1 Reps: 30sec

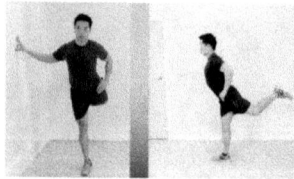 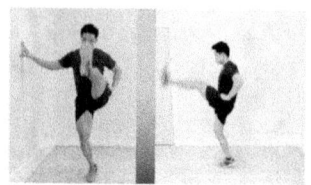

- Stand with feet hip width apart and one hand on a wall to your side.

- Swing your leg forward slightly stretching the back of that leg.

- Swing the same leg back behind your body.

- Repeat the movement gradually increasing the stretch each time.

- Complete all your reps on one side and then on the other.

- This stretch should be started gently and gradually increased.

A6 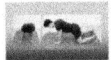 **Moving Cat Stretch**
Sets: 1 Reps: 30sec

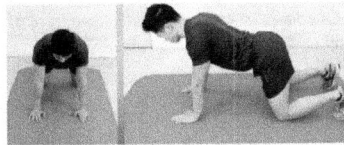 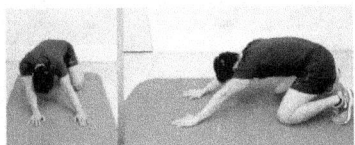

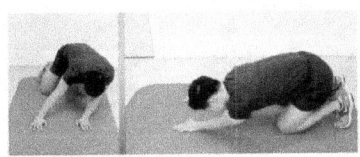

- Start on all fours with a neutral spine.

- Keeping knees on the floor, slowly rock all your weight forwards whilst simultaneously rounding your shoulders.

- From here transfer your weight onto one side (both hands and knees remain in contact with the floor) moving your body back so the weight is now back on your heels. As this is happening pull shoulders down back and down.

- Return to front position, then repeat in opposite direction.

A8 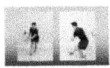 **Dynamic Biceps Femoris Stretch**
Sets: 1 Reps: 30sec

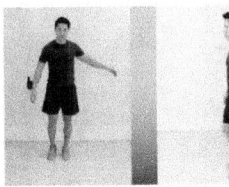 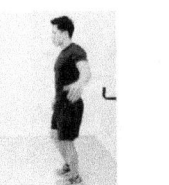 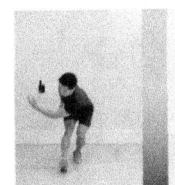 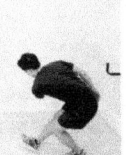

- Take a step forward with one leg and pull up your toes.

- Bend from your hips and reach down to your front foot.

- Go as low as you comfortably can and then twist to the outside. You should feel a stretch at the back on the outside of your front leg.

- Repeat the movement gradually increasing the stretch each time.

- Complete all your reps on one side and then repeat on the other.

A9 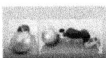 **Dynamic Lat Stretch on Swiss Ball**
Sets: 1 Reps: 30sec

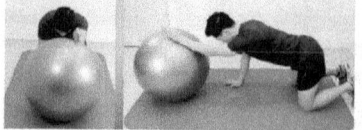
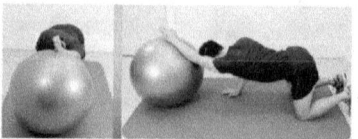

- Take a position on your hands and knees with a Swiss Ball in front of you. Outstretch one arm forward on to the ball with palm facing in.

- Have your head facing the floor and keep your body fixed while moving your arm and the ball forward and slightly in to create a stretch down the side of your back.

A10 **Dynamic Pectoral Stretch**
Sets: 1 Reps: 30sec

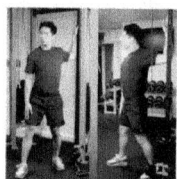
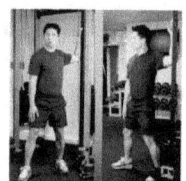

- Stand next to a doorway or corner of a wall. Put the palm of one hand on the wall with a slightly bent elbow. Your arm should be above your shoulder.

- Keeping your hand on the wall, turn away from that arm to stretch your chest.

- Turn back to relieve the stretch and then out into the stretch again.

A11 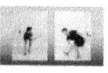 **Dynamic Semimembranosus Stretch**
Sets: 1 Reps: 30sec

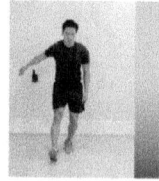
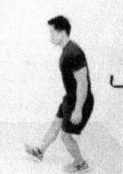
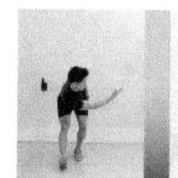
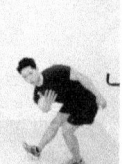

- Take a step forward with one leg and pull up your toes.

- Bend from your hips and reach down to your front foot.

- Go as low as you comfortably can and then twist to the inside. You should feel a stretch at the back on the inside of your front leg.

- Repeat the movement gradually increasing the stretch each time.

- Complete all your reps on one side and then repeat on the other.

Bodybuilding

This is a body part split program similar to those you would find in bodybuilding magazines. It is structured to give you both size and strength with repetition ranges and rest periods to support those goals. It is set up as a five-day program and with a warm-up and cool down each workout will take an average time of an hour.

If you need to lose additional body fat or want cardiovascular training, then you will have to utilize other routines in addition to this program to help support both goals. You could use the running program included as the cardio portion of this program. With the running program included make sure to incorporate adequate rest and recovery and avoid overtraining.

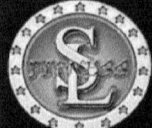
Phase: Bodybuilding - Beginner Week 1 - Program 1

A1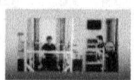

Barbell Back Squat
Sets: 3   Reps: 12-15
Tempo: 3:1:1   Rest: 1:30
Intensity: 15RM

B1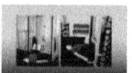

Leg Curl on Suspension Trainer
Sets: 3   Reps: 12-15
Tempo: 1:1:3   Rest: ;1:30
Intensity: 15RM

C1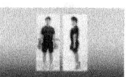

Calf Raise from Floor with Dumbbells
Sets: 3   Reps: 12-15
Tempo: 3:1:1   Rest: 1:30
Intensity: 15RM

D1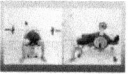

Flat Bench Press - Shoulder Width Grip
Sets: 3   Reps: 12-15
Tempo: 3:1:1   Rest: 1:30
Intensity: 15RM

E1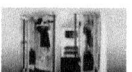

Chin Up - Supinated Shoulder width Grip
Sets: 3   Reps: 12-15
Tempo: 1:1:3   Rest: 1:30
Intensity: 15RM

F1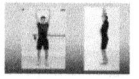

Standing Shoulder Press - Barbell - Shoulder Width Grip
Sets: 3   Reps: 12-15
Tempo: 1:1:3   Rest: 1:30
Intensity: 15RM

G1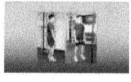

Triceps Extension, High Pulley with Flat Bar
Sets: 3   Reps: 12-15
Tempo: 1:1:3   Rest: 1:30

Intensity: 15RM

H1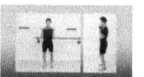

Standing Bicep Curl, Barbell - Medium Grip
Sets: 3   Reps: 12-15
Tempo: 1:1:3   Rest: 1:30
Intensity: 15RM

I1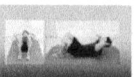

Crunch
Sets: 3   Reps: 12-15
Tempo: 2:1:2   Rest: 1:30
Intensity: 15RM

Phase: Bodybuilding - Beginner Week 1 - Program 2

A1 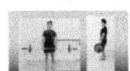 **Dead Lift from Floor Clean Grip**
Sets: 3   Reps: 12-15
Tempo: 1:1:3   Rest: 1:30
Intensity: 15RM

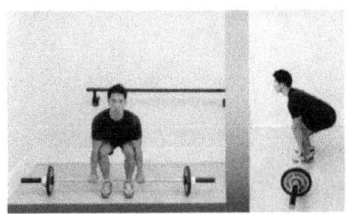 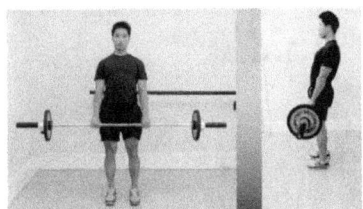

- Start standing with your toes under the bar.

- Lean over, bend your knees and take hold of the bar with your hands a little wider than your knees and palms facing you.

- Push your chest out and hollow your lower back. Gently draw in your tummy with approximately 30% effort.

- Pushing through your feet and keeping your low back hollowed with your chest pushed out, lift the bar until you are standing in an upright position.

- Keeping your low back hollowed with your chest pushed out; lower the bar in a controlled manner down to the floor.

B1 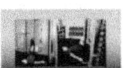 **Leg Curl on Suspension Trainer**
Sets: 3   Reps: 12-15
Tempo: 1:1:3   Rest: 1:30

Intensity: 15RM

68

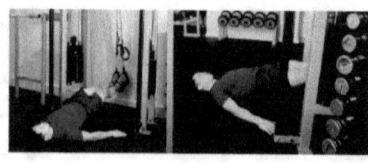 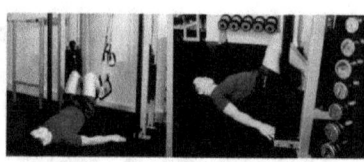

- Lie on your back with your feet hooked in to a suspension trainer.

- Lift your hips up from the ground - they should remain lifted throughout exercise.

- Curl your feet towards your bum.

- Move under control back into the start position.

C1 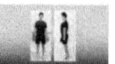 **Calf Raise from Floor with Dumbbells**
Sets: 3   Reps: 12-15
Tempo: 3:1:1   Rest: 1:30
Intensity: 15RM

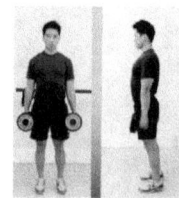 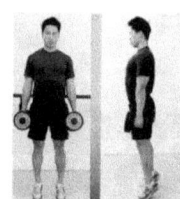

- Take a dumbbell in each hand.

- Stand with your feet a feet hip width apart.

- Keep your chest up and tummy drawn in with 30% effort.

- Working both legs at the same time come right up on your toes as high as you can.

- From the top position lower until your heels are just off the ground a then raise back up again.

D1 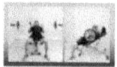 **30° Incline Bench Press - Shoulder Width Grip**
Sets: 3   Reps: 12-15
Tempo: 3:1:1   Rest: 1:30
Intensity: 15RM

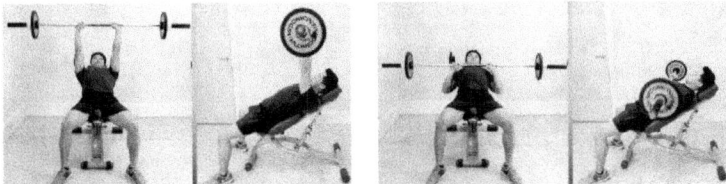

- Lie face up on a 30° inclined bench. Place your hands shoulder width apart on the bar.

- Lower the bar under control down towards your chest.

- As the bar touches your chest lift back up to the top position.

- keep your bum, back and head in contact with the bench at all times.

E1  **Seated Dual Pulley Pull Down - Pronated Grip**
Sets: 3   Reps: 12-15
Tempo: 1:1:3   Rest: 1:30
Intensity: 15RM

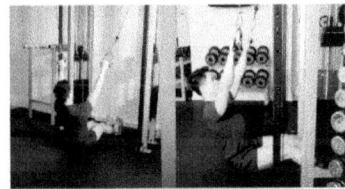 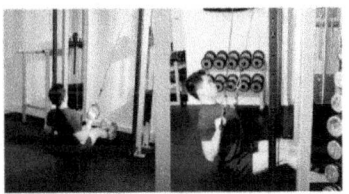

- Sit on the ground with the pulleys set in the top position. Take hold of the handles, one in each hand and with palms facing each away from you.

- Push your chest out, straighten your back, bring your shoulders back and down and lean slightly back.

- Pull the handles towards the outsides of your shoulders. Come back as far as you can while keeping your shoulders back and down.

- Maintaining good posture and control extend your arms to the start position.

F1 **Upright Row with EZ Bar - Medium Grip**
Sets: 3   Reps: 12-1512-15
Tempo: 1:1:3   Rest: 1:30
Intensity: 15RM

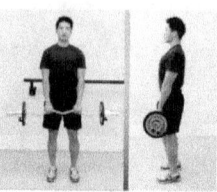 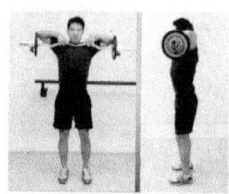

- Stand with your feet hip width apart, tummy gently drawn in with about 30% effort and your shoulders back and down.

- Take a hold of the EZ bar with an overhand grip. Your hands should be on the second V of the bar.

- Standing tall lift the bar to just under your chin. Your elbows should be high and above your hands through the movement.

- Lower back down towards your hips keeping good control of the bar.

G1 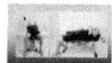 **Lying Triceps Extension with EZ Bar - Narrow Grip**
Sets: 3   Reps: 12-15
Tempo: 3:1:1   Rest: 1:30
Intensity: 15RM

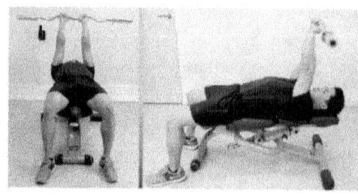 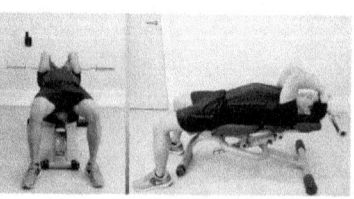

- Lie on the bench facing up. Take the bar on the inside V of the bar with your elbows straight.

- Bend at your elbows lowering the bar to just above your forehead.

- Straighten your elbows back into the start position.

H1 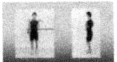 **Standing Bicep Curl, Dumbbells - Neutral to Supinated Grip**
Sets: 3   Reps: 12-15
Tempo: 1:1:3   Rest: 1:30
Intensity: 15RM

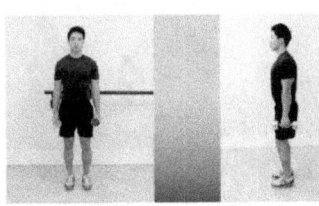 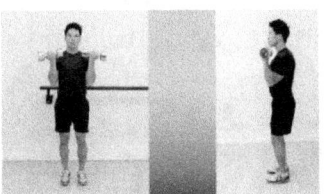

- Stand with feet hip width apart. Take a dumbbell in each hand and turn them so that your palms face each other.

- Start with elbows straight and your wrists firm.

- Keeping your wrists straight, bend at your elbows and twist the dumbbells until your forearms are in contact with the bulge in your biceps and palms are facing up and towards your body. Don't allow your elbows to come forward in the movement.

- Lower under control back down to the straight arm position.

I1 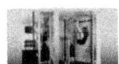 **Hanging Leg Raises**
Sets: 3   Reps: 12-15
Tempo: 1:1:3   Rest: 1:30
Intensity: 15RM

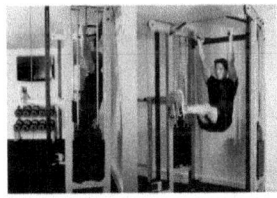 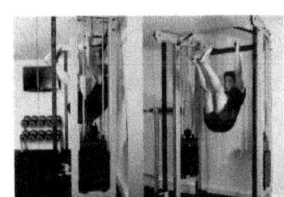

- Hang from a chin up bar.

- Engage your core by drawing your tummy in and pelvic floor (the muscle you would use to stop yourself from peeing) up with 30% effort.

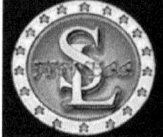

SEMPER LIBERI FITNESS

Phase: Bodybuilding - Beginner Week 1 - Program 2

A1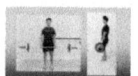
Dead Lift from Floor Clean Grip
Sets: 3 Reps: 12-15
Tempo: 1:1:3 Rest: 1:30
Intensity: 15RM

B1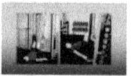
Leg Curl on Suspension Trainer
Sets: 3 Reps: 12-15
Tempo: 1:1:3 Rest: 1:30
Intensity: 15RM

C1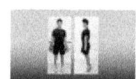
Calf Raise from Floor with Dumbbells
Sets: 3 Reps: 12-15
Tempo: 3:1:1 Rest: 1:30
Intensity: 15RM

D1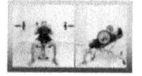
30° Incline Bench Press - Shoulder Width Grip
Sets: 3 Reps: 12-15
Tempo: 3:1:1 Rest: 1:30
Intensity: 15RM

E1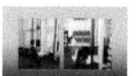
Seated Dual Pulley Pull Down - Pronated Grip
Sets: 3 Reps: 12-15
Tempo: 1:1:3 Rest: 1:30
Intensity: 15RM

F1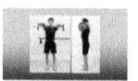
Upright Row with EZ Bar - Medium Grip
Sets: 3 Reps: 12-1512-15
Tempo: 1:1:3 Rest: 1:30
Intensity: 15RM

G1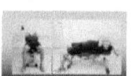
Lying Triceps Extension with EZ Bar - Narrow Grip
Sets: 3 Reps: 12-15
Tempo: 3:1:1 Rest: 1:30
Intensity: 15RM

Intensity: 15RM

I1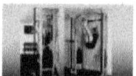
Hanging Leg Raises
Sets: 3 Reps: 12-15
Tempo: 1:1:3 Rest: 1:30
Intensity: 15RM

Phase: Bodybuilding - Beginner Week 1 - Program 1

A1 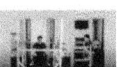 **Barbell Back Squat**
Sets: 3   Reps: 12-15
Tempo: 3:1:1   Rest: 1:30
Intensity: 15RM

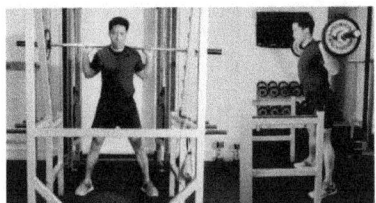 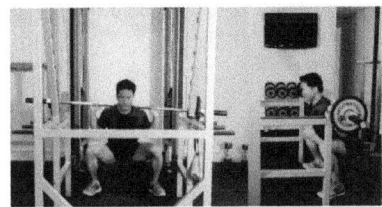

- Stand with your feet parallel and a comfortable distance apart with your weight evenly distributed between both legs.

- Take a barbell on your back, resting it evenly across your shoulders on the cushioned part of your upper back.

- Hold the bar with both hands keeping your elbows directly below your wrists.

- Keeping your chest up, bend at your knees then hips to lower your bum down towards the ground behind you.

- Go as low as you can with control, ideally your hips should go below your knees. Keeping your heels on the ground, push up into the start position.

B1 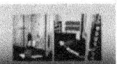 **Leg Curl on Suspension Trainer**
Sets: 3   Reps: 12-15

Tempo: 1:1:3   Rest: ;1:30
Intensity: 15RM

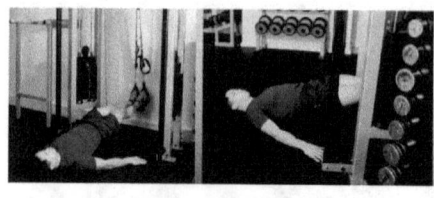 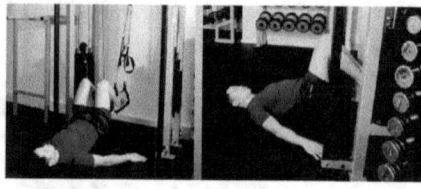

- Lie on your back with your feet hooked in to a suspension trainer.

- Lift your hips up from the ground - they should remain lifted throughout exercise.

- Curl your feet towards your bum.

- Move under control back into the start position.

C1 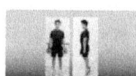 **Calf Raise from Floor with Dumbbells**
Sets: 3　　　　Reps: 12-15
Tempo: 3:1:1　Rest: 1:30
Intensity: 15RM

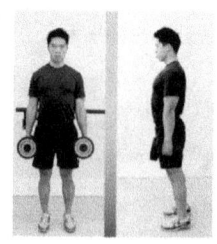 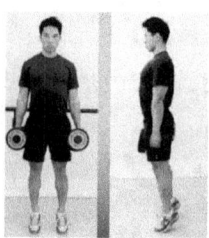

- Take a dumbbell in each hand.

- Stand with your feet a feet hip width apart.

- Keep your chest up and tummy drawn in with 30% effort.

- Working both legs at the same time come right up on your toes as high as you can.

- From the top position lower until your heels are just off the ground a then raise back up again.

D1 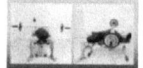 **Flat Bench Press - Shoulder Width Grip**
Sets: 3　　　　Reps: 12-15
Tempo: 3:1:1　Rest: 1:30
Intensity: 15RM

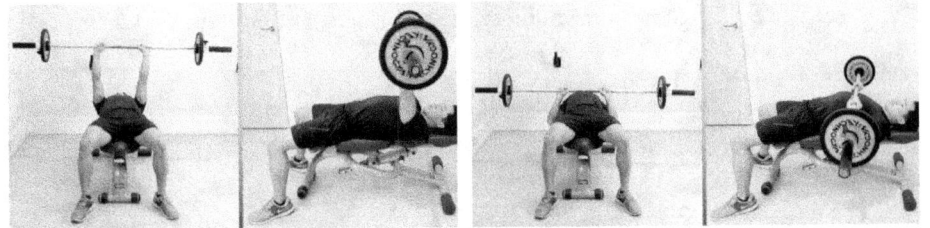

- Lie face up on a bench. Place your hands shoulder width apart on the bar.

- Take the weight and bring it slightly forward so it sits over your chest.

- Lower the bar under control down towards your chest.

- As the bar touches your chest lift back up to the top position.

- keep your bum, back and head in contact with the bench at all times.

E1 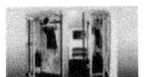 **Chin Up - Supinated Shoulder width Grip**
Sets: 3   Reps: 12-15
Tempo: 1:1:3   Rest: 1:30
Intensity: 15RM

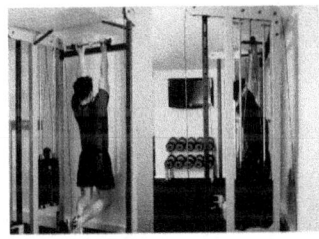   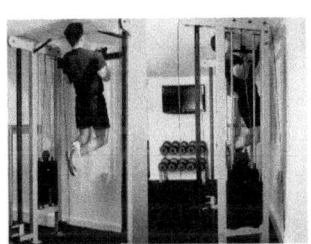

- Stand under the chin up bar at a height where you are able to grip the bar without jumping.

-Take hold of the bar with both hands facing you and shoulder width apart. Bring your shoulder blades back towards each other and down towards your bum.

- Pull yourself up to the top position. Your chin should be above your hands and chest pushed out.

- From the top position, lower your self down under control to the bottom.

F1 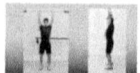 **Standing Shoulder Press - Barbell - Shoulder Width Grip**
Sets: 3   Reps: 12-15
Tempo: 1:1:3   Rest: 1:30
Intensity: 15RM

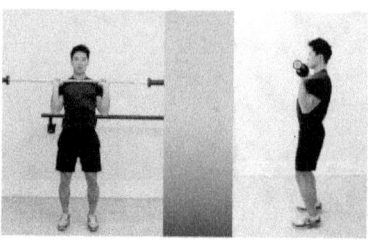 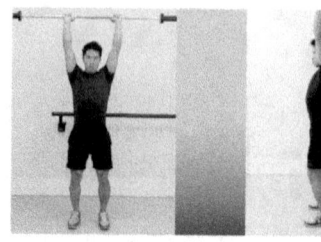

- Stand with your feet hip width apart, tummy gently drawn in with about 30% effort and your shoulders back and down. Take the barbell with a shoulder width grip at shoulder height with your palms facing away from you.

- Keeping your core engaged and body upright push up above your shoulders to a straight arm position.

- Lower under control to the start position.

G1 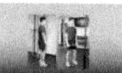 **Triceps Extension, High Pulley with Flat Bar**
Sets: 3   Reps: 12-15
Tempo: 1:1:3   Rest: 1:30
Intensity: 15RM

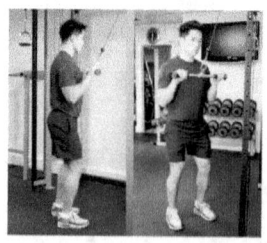 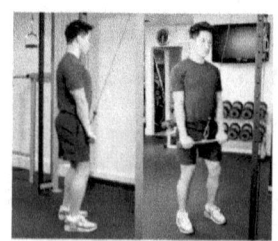

- Stand with feet hip width apart, chest out, chin up and tummy gently drawn in. Take hold of the bar with your palms facing away from you; bring your elbows to your sides.

- Straighten at your elbows moving the bar down towards your hips.

- Then keeping your elbows to your sides bring the bar back up to the start position under control.

H1 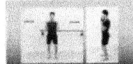 **Standing Bicep Curl, Barbell - Medium Grip**
Sets: 3   Reps: 12-15
Tempo: 1:1:3   Rest: 1:30
Intensity: 15RM

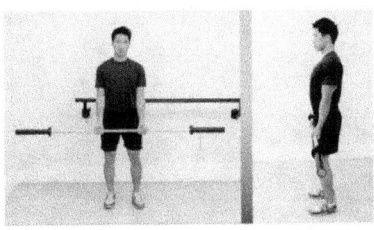 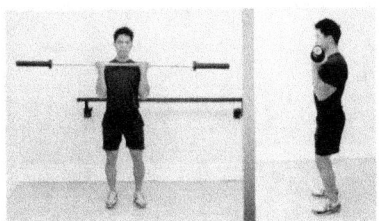

- Stand with feet hip width apart. Take the bar with a shoulder width grip and palms facing away from your body.

- Start with elbows straight and your wrists firm.

- Keeping your wrists straight, bend at your elbows until your forearms are in contact with the bulge in your biceps. Don't allow your elbows to come forward in the movement.

- Lower under control back down to the straight arm position.

I1 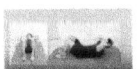 **Crunch**
Sets: 3   Reps: 12-15
Tempo: 2:1:2   Rest: 1:30
Intensity: 15RM

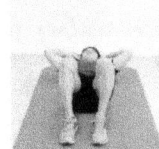 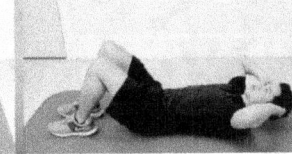 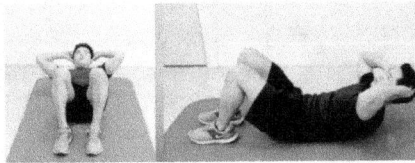

- Engage your core by drawing your tummy in and pelvic floor muscle (the muscle you would use to stop yourself from peeing) up with 30% effort.

- Put your tongue on the roof of your mouth, this will stop the muscles in the front of your neck overworking.

- Tuck your chin gently towards your chest and lift your shoulders and shoulder blades off the mat. Keeping your feet on the ground and core engaged; lift your torso as far towards your knees as you can.

- Lower back down under control so that your shoulder blades are once again on the mat.

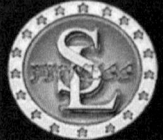

Phase: Bodybuilding - Beginner Week 1 - Program 3

A1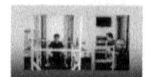
Barbell Back Squat
Sets: 3 Reps: 12-15
Tempo: 3:1:1 Rest: 1:30
Intensity: 15RM

B1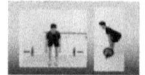
Romanian Deadlift Clean Grip
Sets: 3 Reps: 12-15
Tempo: 3:1:1 Rest: 1:30
Intensity: 15RM

C1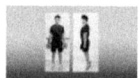
Calf Raise from Floor with Dumbbells
Sets: 3 Reps: 12-15
Tempo: 3:1:1 Rest: 1:30
Intensity: 15RM

D1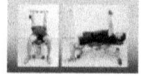
Flat Chest press with Dumbells - Pronated Grip
Sets: 3 Reps: 12-15
Tempo: 3:1:1 Rest: 1:30
Intensity: 15RM

E1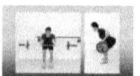
Bent over Row, Barbell - Clean Grip
Sets: 3 Reps: 12-15
Tempo: 3:1:1 Rest: 1:30
Intensity: 15RM

F1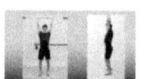
Standing Shoulder Press - Barbell - Shoulder Width Grip
Sets: 3 Reps: 12-15
Tempo: 1:1:3 Rest: 1:30
Intensity: 15RM

G1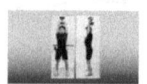
Overhead Triceps Extension with Single Dumbbell
Sets: 3 Reps: 12-15
Tempo: 1:1:3 Rest: 1:30
Intensity: 15RM

H1
Sets: 3 Reps: 12-15
Tempo: 1:1:3 Rest: 1:30
Intensity: 15RM

I1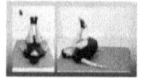
Lying Garhammers
Sets: 3 Reps: 12-15
Tempo: 1:1:3 Rest: 1:30
Intensity: 15RM

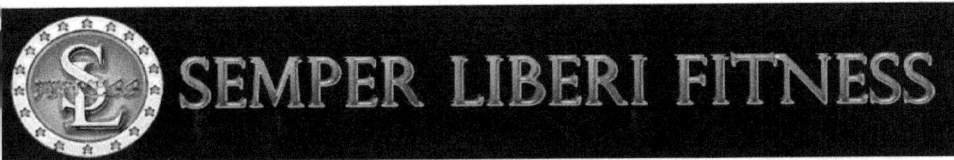
Phase: Bodybuilding - Beginner Week 1 - Program 3

A1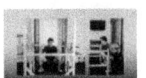
Barbell Back Squat
Sets: 3   Reps: 12-15
Tempo: 3:1:1   Rest: 1:30
Intensity: 15RM

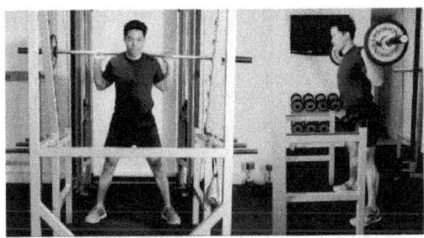 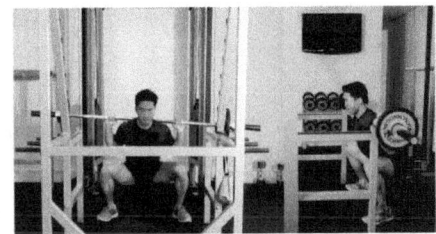

- Stand with your feet parallel and a comfortable distance apart with your weight evenly distributed between both legs.

- Take a barbell on your back, resting it evenly across your shoulders on the cushioned part of your upper back.

- Hold the bar with both hands keeping your elbows directly below your wrists.

- Keeping your chest up, bend at your knees then hips to lower your bum down towards the ground behind you.

- Go as low as you can with control, ideally your hips should go below your knees. Keeping your heels on the ground, push up into the start position.

B1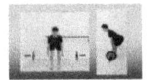
Romanian Deadlift Clean Grip
Sets: 3   Reps: 12-15

Tempo: 3:1:1   Rest: 1:30
Intensity: 15RM

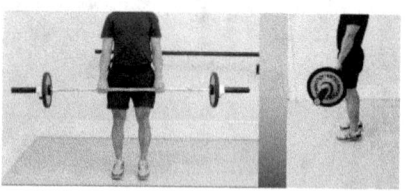 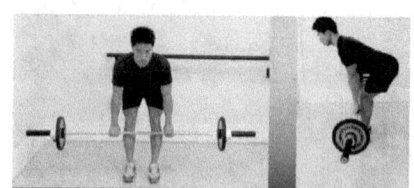

- Start standing with your toes under the bar.

- Lean over and take hold of the bar with your hands a little wider than your knees and palms facing you.

- Push your chest out and hollow your lower back. Gently draw in your tummy with approximately 30% effort.

- With your knees nearly straight (with just a little give) and keeping your low back hollowed with your chest pushed out, lift the bar and thrust your hips forward until you are standing in an upright position.

- Keeping your low back hollowed with your chest pushed out, lower the bar in a controlled manner until you feel a stretch in the back of your legs.

- Lift the bar again.

C1 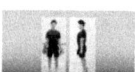 **Calf Raise from Floor with Dumbbells**

Sets: 3   Reps: 12-15
Tempo: 3:1:1   Rest: 1:30
Intensity: 15RM

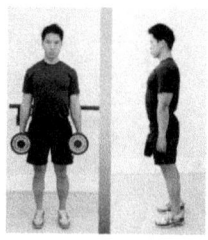 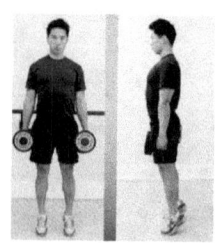

- Take a dumbbell in each hand.

- Stand with your feet a feet hip width apart.

- Keep your chest up and tummy drawn in with 30% effort.

- Working both legs at the same time come right up on your toes as high as you can.

- From the top position lower until your heels are just off the ground a then raise back up again.

D1 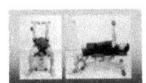 **Flat Chest press with Dumbells - Pronated Grip**
Sets: 3   Reps: 12-15
Tempo: 3:1:1   Rest: 1:30
Intensity: 15RM

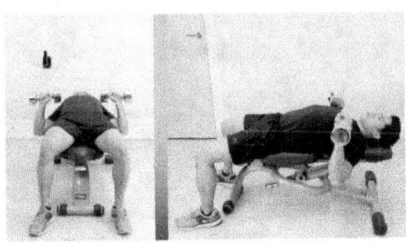 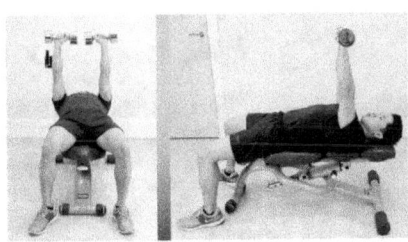

- Lie face up on a bench with a dumbbell in each hand and palms facing your feet.

- Start in the bottom position and extend your arms bringing your hands in front of your shoulders with elbows straight.

- Lower back down under control to a position just outside your body and as low as you can go before pushing back up again.

- Keep your bum, back and head in contact with the bench at all times.

E1   **Bent over Row, Barbell - Clean Grip**

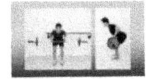 Sets: 3   Reps: 12-15
Tempo: 3:1:1   Rest: 1:30
Intensity: 15RM

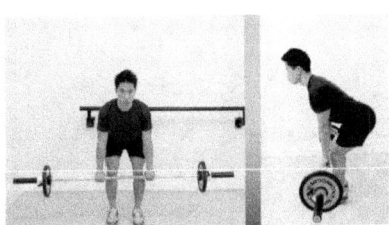 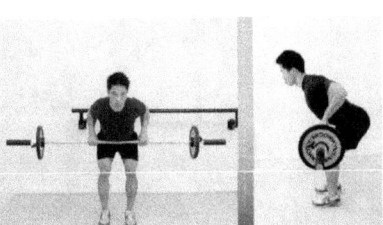

- Keeping your shoulders back and down pull the bar in towards your bottom ribs.

- Lower the bar under control back down to the starting position.

F1 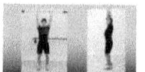 **Standing Shoulder Press - Barbell - Shoulder Width Grip**
Sets: 3   Reps: 12-15
Tempo: 1:1:3   Rest: 1:30
Intensity: 15RM

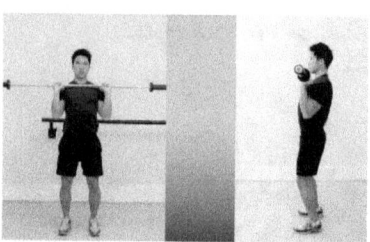 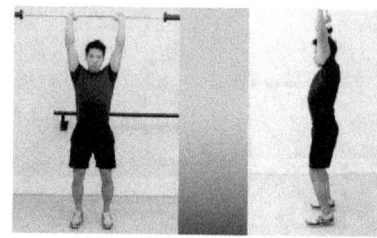

- Stand with your feet hip width apart, tummy gently drawn in with about 30% effort and your shoulders back and down. Take the barbell with a shoulder width grip at shoulder height with your palms facing away from you.

- Keeping your core engaged and body upright push up above your shoulders to a straight arm position.

- Lower under control to the start position.

G1 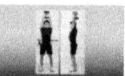 **Overhead Triceps Extension with Single Dumbbell**
Sets: 3   Reps: 12-15
Tempo: 1:1:3   Rest: 1:30
Intensity: 15RM

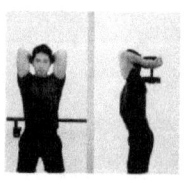 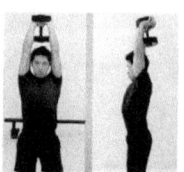

83

- Stand with feet hip width apart, chest out, chin up and tummy gently drawn in.

- Take hold of a dumbbell in both hands.

- Start with elbows bent overhead and hands behind your back.

- Straighten your elbows to bring the dumbbell straight up above your head.

- Bend your elbow to return under control to the start position.

H1 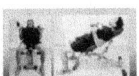 **Seated Incline Hammer Curl**
Sets: 3   Reps: 12-15
Tempo: 1:1:3   Rest: 1:30
Intensity: 15RM

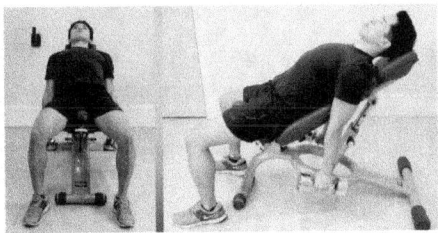 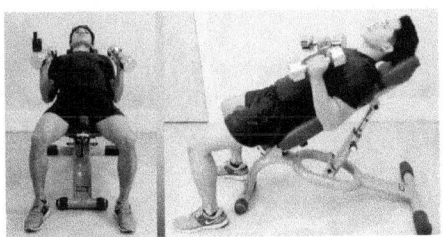

- Sit with the bench in an incline position and your arms down to your sides. Take hold of the dumbbells with your palms facing each other and your elbows straight.

- Keeping your elbows back and wrists firm, curl the weight up until your forearms touch the bulge in your biceps.

- Lower under control back down to the straight arm position.

I1 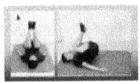 **Lying Garhammers**
Sets: 3   Reps: 12-15
Tempo: 1:1:3   Rest: 1:30
Intensity: 15RM

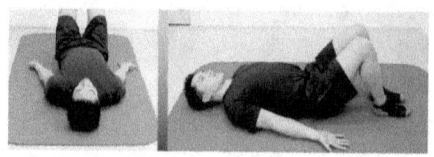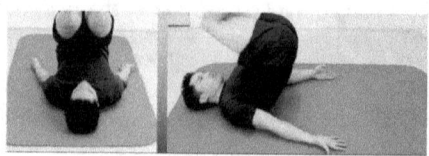

- Lie on your back with knees bent and palms facing up.

- Engage your core by drawing your tummy in and pelvic floor (the muscle you would use to stop yourself from peeing) up with 30% effort.

- Put your tongue on the roof of your mouth, this will stop the muscles in the front of your neck overworking.

- Lift your legs out above your hips, thrust your hips straight up lifting your lower spine off the mat.

- Slowly lower back down under good control until your feet are just above the ground. Keep your head and shoulder blades on the mat throughout the movement.

Circuit Training

This is a sample program that is designed from a circuit training model. It is set up with similar principles to P90X and will give you an idea of what the program entails. I have not tried the newer versions of P90X, and I do not know how they relate to the program I participated in, but I thought it was an excellent program, and if you enjoy the circuit training program that is included here, P90X may be a great fitness solution for you.

Phase: Circuit 1 - Program 1

A1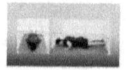
Press Up Flat
Sets: 2   Reps: 12-15
Tempo: Fast Intensity: 15RM

A2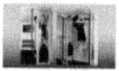
Pull Up - Shoulder Width Grip
Sets: 2   Reps: 12-15
Tempo: Fast Intensity: 15RM

B1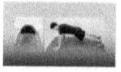
Press Up - Side to Side
Sets: 2   Reps: 12-15
Tempo: Fast Intensity: 15RM

B2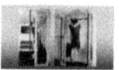
Pull Up, Side to Side - Wide Grip
Sets: 2   Reps: 12-15
Tempo: Fast Intensity: 15RM

C1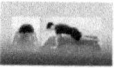
Press Up - Zig Zag
Sets: 2   Reps: 12-15
Tempo: Fast Intensity: 15RM

C2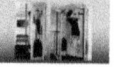
Pull Up - Narrow Grip
Sets: 2   Reps: 12-15
Tempo: Fast Intensity: 15RM

D1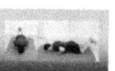
Press Up on Knees - Narrow Grip
Sets: 2   Reps: 12-15
Tempo: Fast Intensity: 15RM

D2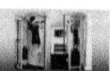
Chin Up - Neutral Grip
Sets: 2   Reps: 12-15
Tempo: Fast Intensity: 15RM

E1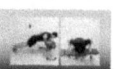
Press Up to Bench
Sets: 2   Reps: 12-15

E2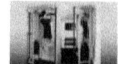
Chin Up - Supinated Narrow Grip
Sets: 2   Reps: 12-15
Tempo: Fast Intensity: 15RM

Phase: Circuit 1 - Program 1

A1 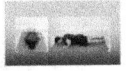 **Press Up Flat**
Sets: 2   Reps: 12-15
Tempo: Fast Intensity: 15RM

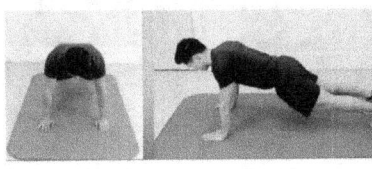 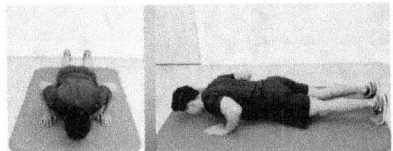

- Come down so that your hands and feet are on the floor.

- Place your hands a little wider than shoulder width apart.

- Position your hips to form a straight line from your heels to your head.

- Gently draw in your tummy using roughly 30% effort.

- Bend your elbows lowering your body toward the ground. Keep your elbows at about 45 degrees from the sides of your body.

- You should come down so that your chest is between your hands.

- Lower until your chest is a small fist away from the ground and then push back up to the start position.

A2 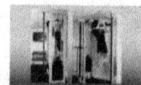 **Pull Up - Shoulder Width Grip**
Sets: 2   Reps: 12-15
Tempo: Fast Intensity: 15RM

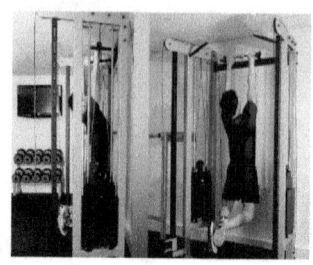 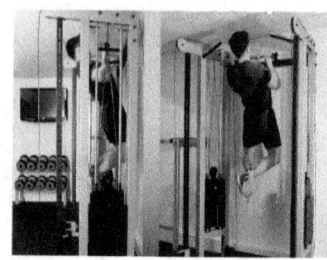

- Stand under the chin up bar at a height where you are able to grip the bar without jumping.

-Take hold of the bar with both hands facing away from you and shoulder width apart. Bring your shoulder blades back towards each other and down towards your bum.

- Pull yourself up to the top position. Your chin should be above your hands and chest pushed out.

- From the top position, lower your self down under control to the bottom.

B1 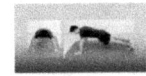 **Press Up - Side to Side**
Sets: 2   Reps: 12-15
Tempo: Fast Intensity: 15RM

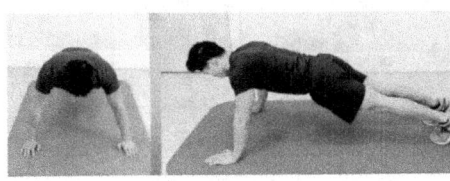 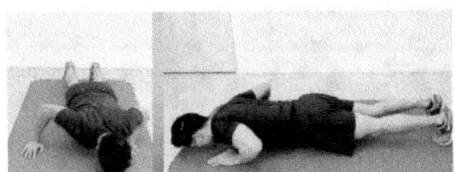

- Come down so that your hands and feet are on the floor.

- Place your hands a little wider than shoulder width apart.

- Position your hips to form a straight line from your heels to your head.

- Gently draw in your tummy using roughly 30% effort.

- Bend your elbows and lower your body toward one arm and the ground.

- You should come down so that your chest is between your hands and parallel to the ground.

- Lower until your chest is a small fist away from the ground and then push back up to the start position.

- Then bend your elbows again to lower your body over towards the other arm.

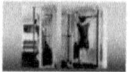 **B2**   **Pull Up, Side to Side - Wide Grip**
Sets: 2   Reps: 12-15
Tempo: Fast Intensity: 15RM

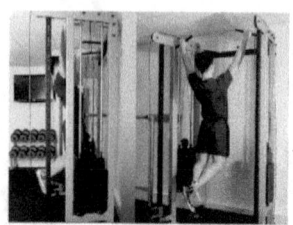 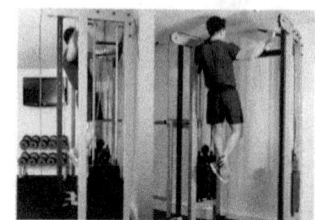

- Stand under the chin up bar at a height where you are able to grip the bar without jumping.

-Take hold of the bar with both hands facing away from you and 1 ½ times shoulder width apart. Bring your shoulder blades back towards each other and down towards your bum.

- Pull yourself up towards one hand. Your chin should be above your hands and chest pushed out.

- Lower your self down under control to the bottom and then repeat going up towards the other hand.

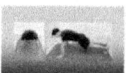 **C1**   **Press Up - Zig Zag**
Sets: 2   Reps: 12-15
Tempo: Fast Intensity: 15RM

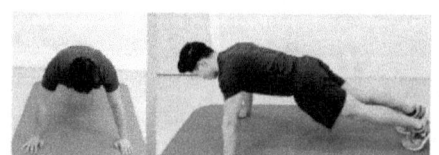 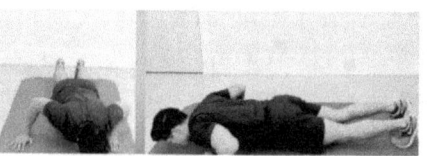

- Come down so that your hands and feet are on the floor.

- Place your hands a little wider than shoulder width apart.

- Position your hips to form a straight line from your heels to your head.

- Gently draw in your tummy using roughly 30% effort.

- Bend your elbows and lower your body toward one arm and the ground.

- You should come down so that your chest is between your hands and parallel to the ground.

- Lower until your chest is a small fist away from the ground and then push your torso across towards your other arm.

- Push up in to the start position.

C2 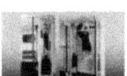 **Pull Up - Narrow Grip**
Sets: 2   Reps: 12-15
Tempo: Fast Intensity: 15RM

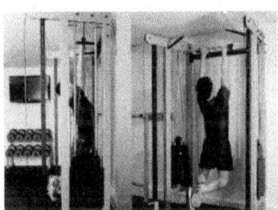 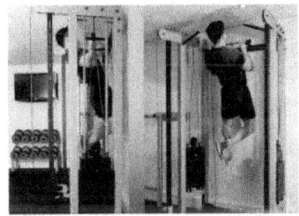

- Stand under the chin up bar at a height where you are able to grip the bar without jumping.

-Take hold of the bar with both hands facing away from you and inside shoulder width apart. Bring your shoulder blades back towards each other and down towards your bum.

- Pull yourself up to the top position. Your chin should be above your hands and chest pushed out.

- From the top position, lower your self down under control to the bottom.

D1 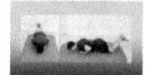 **Press Up on Knees - Narrow Grip**
Sets: 2   Reps: 12-15
Tempo: Fast Intensity: 15RM

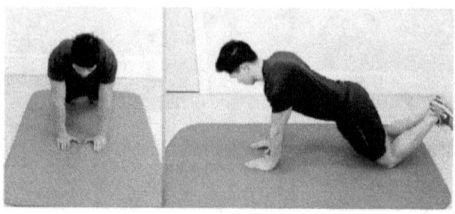 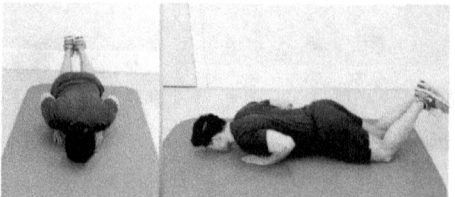

- Come down so that your hands and knees are on the floor.

- Place your hands about two thumbs apart.

- Gently draw in your tummy using approximately 30% effort.

- Bend your elbows lowering your body toward the ground. Keep your elbows close to the sides of your body.

- You should come down so that your chest is between your hands.

- Lower until your chest is a small fist away from the ground and then push back up to the start position.

D2 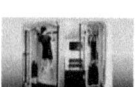 **Chin Up - Neutral Grip**
Sets: 2   Reps: 12-15
Tempo: Fast Intensity: 15RM

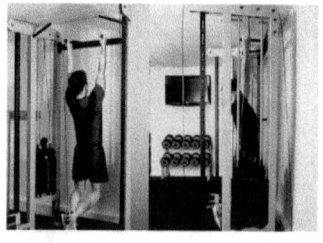 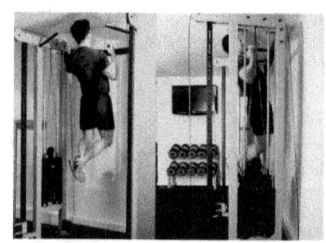

- Stand under the chin up bar at a height where you are able to grip the bar without jumping.

-Take hold of the bar with both hands facing each other. Bring your shoulder blades back towards each other and down towards your bum.

- Pull yourself up to the top position. Your chin should be above your hands and chest pushed out.

- From the top position, lower your self down under control to the bottom.

E1 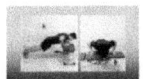 **Press Up to Bench**
Sets: 2   Reps: 12-15
Tempo: Fast Intensity: 15RM

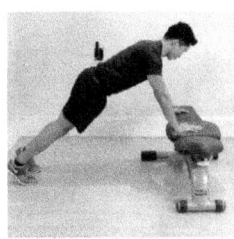 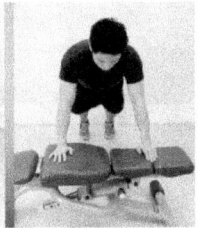 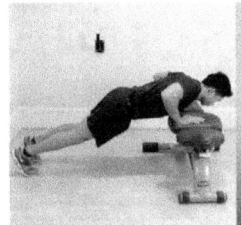 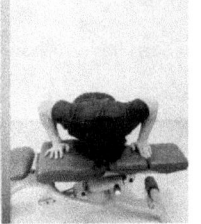

- Come down so that your feet are on the floor and hands on a bench.

- Place your hands a little wider than shoulder width apart.

- Position your hips to form a straight line from your heels to your head.

- Gently draw in your tummy using roughly 30% effort.

- Bend your elbows lowering your body toward the ground. Keep your elbows at 45 degrees from the sides of your body.

- You should come down so that your chest is between your hands.

- Lower until your chest is a small fist away from the step and then push back up to the start position.

E2   **Chin Up - Supinated Narrow Grip**
Sets: 2   Reps: 12-15

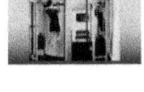   Tempo: Fast Intensity: 15RM

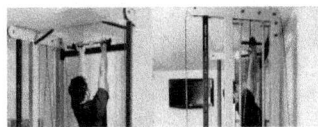   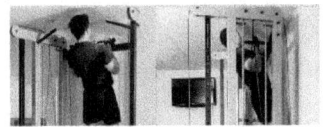

- Stand under the chin up bar at a height where you are able to grip the bar without jumping.

-Take hold of the bar with both hands facing you and inside shoulder width apart. Bring your shoulder blades back towards each other and down towards your bum.

- Pull yourself up to the top position. Your chin should be above your hands and chest pushed out.

- From the top position, lower your self down under control to the bottom.

Phase: Circuit 1 - Program 2

A1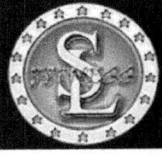
Seated Shoulder Press - Dumbbells - Supinated to Pronated Grip
Sets: 2   Reps: 12-15
Tempo: Fast Intensity: 15RM

A2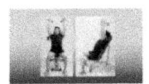
Incline Lying Triceps Extension with Dumbbells - Neutral Grip
Sets: 2   Reps: 12-15
Tempo: Fast Intensity: 15RM

A3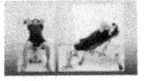
Standing Bicep Curl, Dumbbells - Supinated Grip
Sets: 2   Reps: 12-15
Tempo: Fast Intensity: 15RM

B1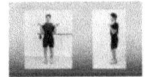
Seated Shoulder Press - Dumbbells - Pronated Grip
Sets: 2   Reps: 12-15
Tempo: Fast Intensity: 15RM

B2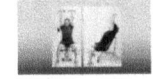
Lying Triceps Extension with Dumbbells - Neutral Grip
Sets: 2   Reps: 12-15
Tempo: Fast Intensity: 15RM

B3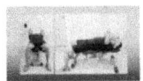
Standing Bicep Curl, Dumbbells - Neutral to Supinated Grip
Sets: 2   Reps: 12-15
Tempo: Fast Intensity: 15RM

C1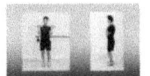
Lateral Raise - Dumbbells
Sets: 2   Reps: 12-15
Tempo: Fast Intensity: 15RM

C2
Overhead Triceps Extension with Dumbbells - Neutral Grip
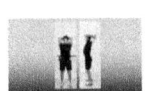
Sets: 2   Reps: 12-15
Tempo: Fast Intensity: 15RM

C3 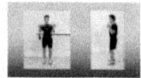 **Standing Bicep Curl, Dumbbells - Pronated Grip**
Sets: 2   Reps: 12-15
Tempo: Fast Intensity: 15RM

D1 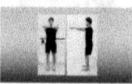 **Front Raise - Dumbbells - Pronated Grip**
Sets: 2   Reps: 12-15
Tempo: Fast Intensity: 15RM

D2 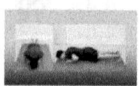 **Press Up with Narrow Grip**
Sets: 2   Reps: 12-15
Tempo: Fast Intensity: 15RM

D3 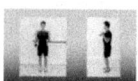 **Standing Hammer Curl**
Sets: 2   Reps: 12-15
Tempo: Fast Intensity: 15RM

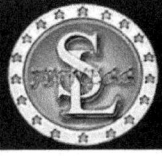

SEMPER LIBERI FITNESS

Phase: Circuit 1 - Program 2

A1 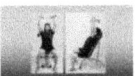 **Seated Shoulder Press - Dumbbells - Supinated to Pronated Grip**
Sets: 2   Reps: 12-15
Tempo: Fast Intensity: 15RM

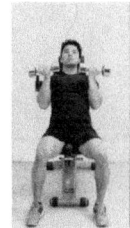 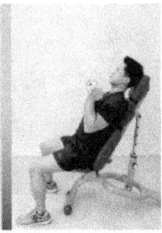 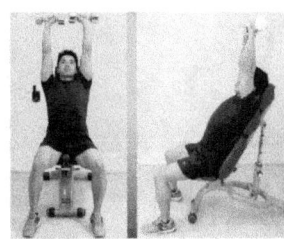

- Sit with your back supported on the rest. Lift the dumbbells to shoulder height with your palms facing your chest.

- Without arching your back push up above your shoulders to a straight arm position. While pushing the dumbbells, twist so that your palms face away from you.

- Lower under control to the start position.

A2 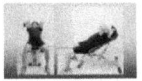 **Incline Lying Triceps Extension with Dumbbells - Neutral Grip**
Sets: 2   Reps: 12-15
Tempo: Fast Intensity: 15RM

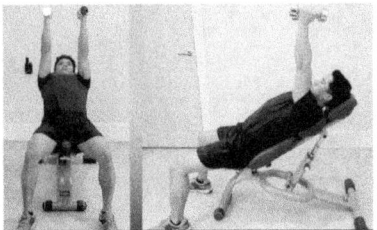 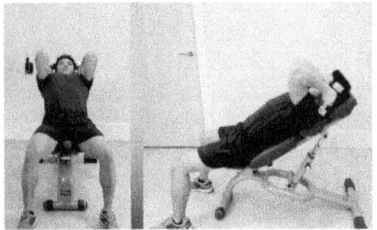

- Lie on an incline bench facing up. Take a dumbbell in each hand with your palms facing each other.

- Bend at your elbows lowering the dumbbells over your shoulders to just above the bench.

- Straighten your elbows back into the start position.

A3 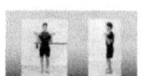 **Standing Bicep Curl, Dumbbells - Supinated Grip**
Sets: 2   Reps: 12-15
Tempo: Fast Intensity: 15RM

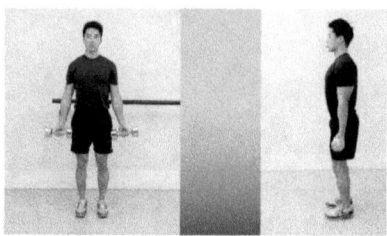 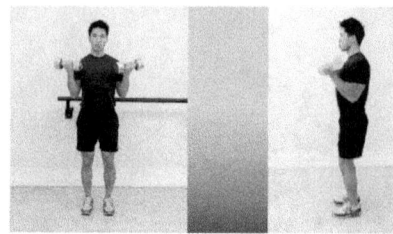

- Stand with feet hip width apart. Take a dumbbell in each hand and turn them so that your palms face away from your body.

- Start with elbows straight and your wrists firm.

- Keeping your wrists straight, bend at your elbows until your forearms are in contact with the bulge in your biceps. Don't allow your elbows to come forward in the movement.

- Lower under control back down to the straight arm position.

B1 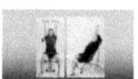 **Seated Shoulder Press - Dumbbells - Pronated Grip**
Sets: 2   Reps: 12-15
Tempo: Fast Intensity: 15RM

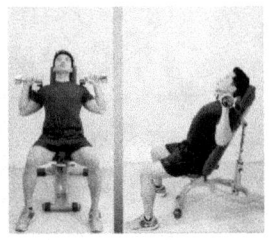 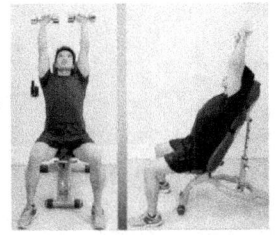

- Sit with your back supported on the rest. Lift the dumbbells to shoulder height with your palms facing forward.

- Without arching your back push up above your shoulders to a straight arm position.

- Lower under control to the start position.

B2 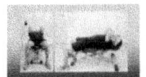 **Lying Triceps Extension with Dumbbells - Neutral Grip**
Sets: 2   Reps: 12-15
Tempo: Fast Intensity: 15RM

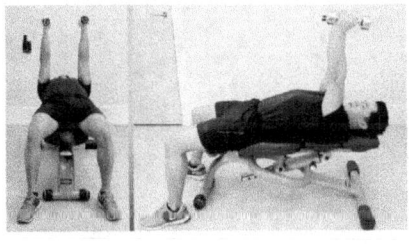 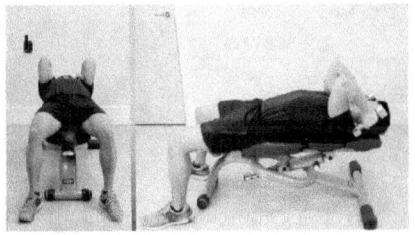

- Lie on the bench facing up. Take a dumbbell in each hand with your palms facing each other.

- Bend at your elbows lowering the dumbbells over your shoulders to just above the bench.

- Straighten your elbows back into the start position.

B3 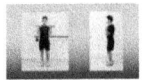 **Standing Bicep Curl, Dumbbells - Neutral to Supinated Grip**
Sets: 2   Reps: 12-15
Tempo: Fast Intensity: 15RM

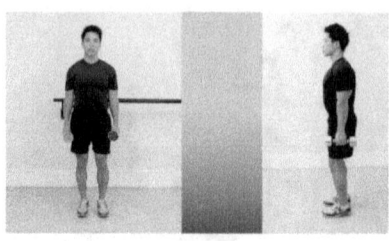
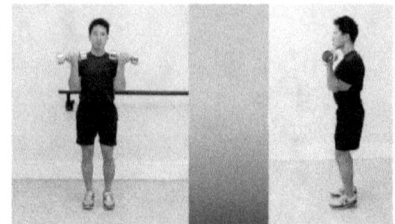

- Stand with feet hip width apart. Take a dumbbell in each hand and turn them so that your palms face each other.

- Start with elbows straight and your wrists firm.

- Keeping your wrists straight, bend at your elbows and twist the dumbbells until your forearms are in contact with the bulge in your biceps and palms are facing up and towards your body. Don't allow your elbows to come forward in the movement.

- Lower under control back down to the straight arm position.

C1 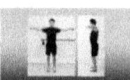 **Lateral Raise - Dumbbells**
Sets: 2   Reps: 12-15
Tempo: Fast Intensity: 15RM

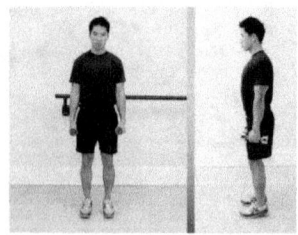
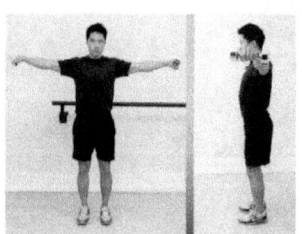

- Stand with your feet hip width apart, tummy gently drawn in with about 30% effort and your shoulders back and down. Take a dumbbell in each hand.

- Start with the dumbbells to your sides.

- Raise the dumbbells out to your sides up to shoulder height.

- Lower under control to the start position.

C2 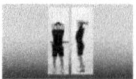 **Overhead Triceps Extension with Dumbbells - Neutral Grip**
Sets: 2   Reps: 12-15
Tempo: Fast Intensity: 15RM

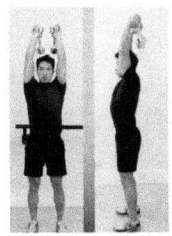 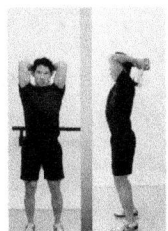

- Stand with feet hip width apart, chest out, chin up and tummy gently drawn in.

- Take hold of a dumbbell in each hand.

- Start with elbows bent overhead and hands behind your back.

- Straighten your elbows to bring the dumbbells straight up above your head.

- Bend your elbows to return under control to the start position.

C3 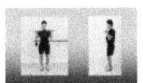 **Standing Bicep Curl, Dumbbells - Pronated Grip**
Sets: 2   Reps: 12-15
Tempo: Fast Intensity: 15RM

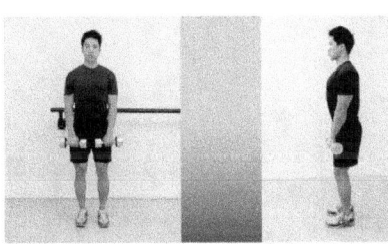 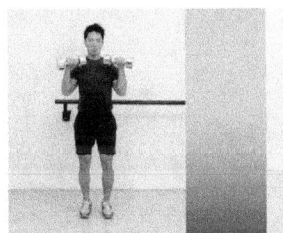 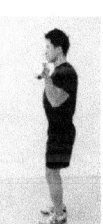

- Stand with feet hip width apart. Take a dumbbell in each hand and turn them so that your palms face your body.

- Start with elbows straight and your wrists firm.

- Keeping your wrists straight, bend at your elbows until your forearms are in contact with the bulge in your biceps. Don't allow your elbows to come forward in the movement.

- Lower under control back down to the straight arm position.

D1 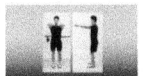 **Front Raise - Dumbbells - Pronated Grip**
Sets: 2   Reps: 12-15
Tempo: Fast Intensity: 15RM

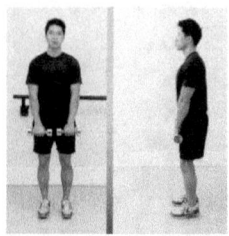 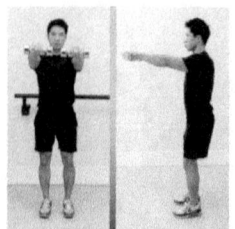

- Stand with your feet hip width apart, tummy gently drawn in with about 30% effort and your shoulders back and down. Take a dumbbell in each hand with your hands in front of your body and palms facing you.

- Keeping your core engaged, body upright and elbows straight, raise the dumbbells in front of your body to shoulder height. Your palms should be facing the floor at the top position.

- Lower under control to the start position.

D2 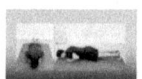 **Press Up with Narrow Grip**
Sets: 2   Reps: 12-15
Tempo: Fast Intensity: 15RM

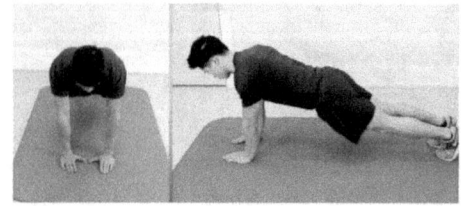 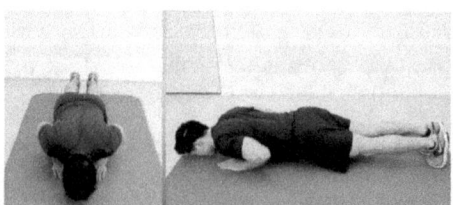

- Place your hands on the floor roughly 2 thumbs apart.

- Gently draw in your tummy using roughly 30% effort.

- Bend your elbows lowering your body toward the ground. Keep your elbows close to your body.

- Lower until your chest is a small fist away from the ground and then push back up to the start position.

D3 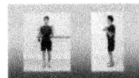 **Standing Hammer Curl**
Sets: 2   Reps: 12-15
Tempo: Fast Intensity: 15RM

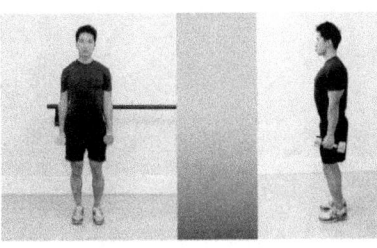 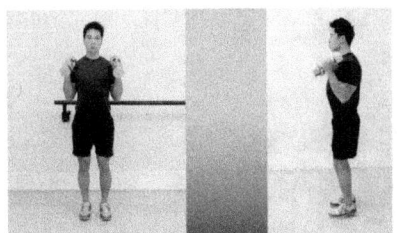

- Stand with feet hip width apart. Take a dumbbell in each hand and turn them so that your palms face each other.

- Start with elbows straight and your wrists firm.

- Keeping your wrists straight, bend at your elbows until your forearms are in contact with the bulge in your biceps. Don't allow your elbows to come forward in the movement.

- Lower under control back down to the straight arm position.

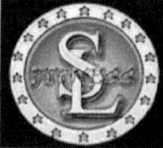

SEMPER LIBERI FITNESS

Phase: Circuit 1 - Program 3

A1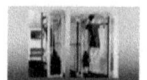
Pull Up - Wide Grip
Sets: 2   Reps: 12-15
Tempo: Fast Intensity: 15RM

A2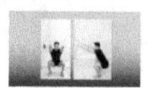
Body Weight Squat
Sets: 2   Reps: 12-15
Tempo: Fast Intensity: 15RM

B1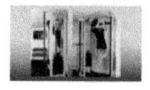
Pull Up - Shoulder Width Grip
Sets: 2   Reps: 12-15
Tempo: Fast Intensity: 15RM

B2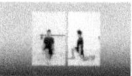
90° Lunge, Flat with Dumbbells
Sets: 2   Reps: 12-15
Tempo: Fast Intensity: 15RM

C1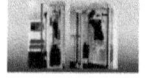
Pull Up - Narrow Grip
Sets: 2   Reps: 12-15
Tempo: Fast Intensity: 15RM

C2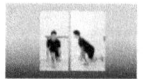
Single Leg Dead Lift with Dumbbells
Sets: 2   Reps: 12-15
Tempo: Fast Intensity: 15RM

D1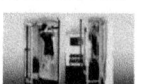
Chin Up - Supinated Shoulder width Grip
Sets: 2   Reps: 12-15
Tempo: Fast Intensity: 15RM

D2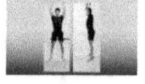
Squat Jump
Sets: 2   Reps: 12-15
Tempo: Fast Intensity: 15RM

E1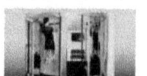
Chin Up - Neutral Grip
Sets: 2   Reps: 12-15

Tempo: Fast Intensity: 15RM

E2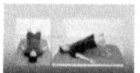
Supine Bridge
Sets: 2   Reps: 12-15
Tempo: Fast Intensity: 15RM

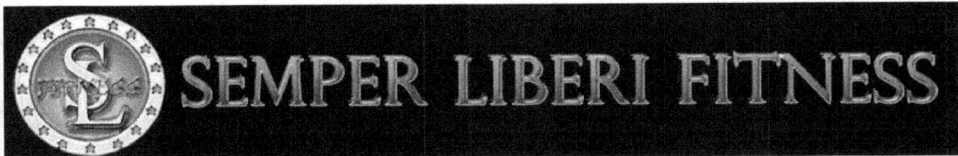

Phase: Circuit 1 - Program 3

A1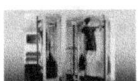

Pull Up - Wide Grip
Sets: 2   Reps: 12-15
Tempo: Fast Intensity: 15RM

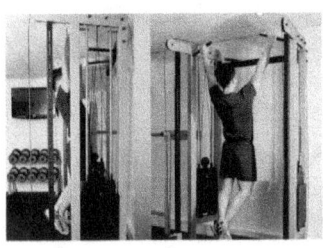 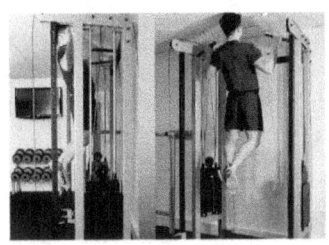

- Stand under the chin up bar at a height where you are able to grip the bar without jumping.

-Take hold of the bar with both hands facing away from you and 1 ½ times shoulder width apart. Bring your shoulder blades back towards each other and down towards your bum.

- Pull yourself up to the top position. Your chin should be above your hands and chest pushed out.

- From the top position, lower your self down under control to the bottom.

A2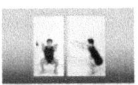

Body Weight Squat
Sets: 2   Reps: 12-15
Tempo: Fast Intensity: 15RM

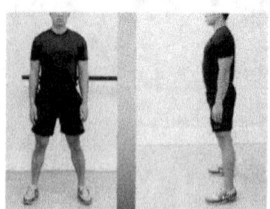 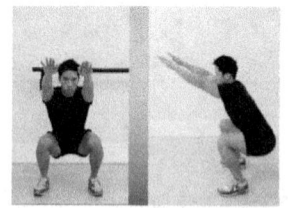

- Stand with your feet parallel and a comfortable distance apart with your weight evenly distributed between both legs.

- Keeping your chest up, bend at your knees then hips to lower your bum down towards the ground behind you.

- Go as low as you can with control, ideally your hips should go below your knees.

- Keeping your weight evenly distributed, push up as fast as you can.

B1 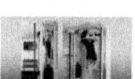 **Pull Up - Shoulder Width Grip**
Sets: 2   Reps: 12-15
Tempo: Fast Intensity: 15RM

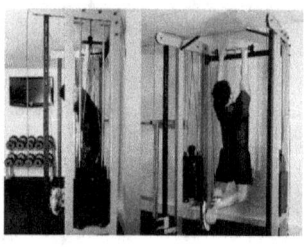 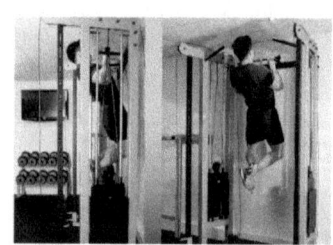

- Stand under the chin up bar at a height where you are able to grip the bar without jumping.

-Take hold of the bar with both hands facing away from you and shoulder width apart. Bring your shoulder blades back towards each other and down towards your bum.

- Pull yourself up to the top position. Your chin should be above your hands and chest pushed out.

- From the top position, lower your self down under control to the bottom.

B2 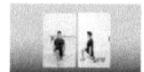 **90° Lunge, Flat with Dumbbells**
Sets: 2   Reps: 12-15

Tempo: Fast Intensity: 15RM

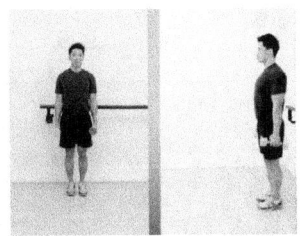 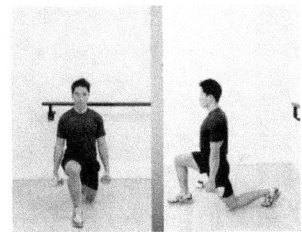

- Take a dumbbell in each hand.

- Push your chest up and draw in your tummy with 30% effort. Step forward approximately 1 ½ times natural stride length.

- Putting your weight on your front leg lower yourself straight down keeping your front knee behind your toes.

- Coming down there should be approximately a 90 degree angle at the back of both knees. Your back heel should come off the ground.

- From the bottom position push back up with your weight coming through your front foot. Your front foot should come back to the start position of the exercise.

- Keep your head and chest upright with your hips level and forward facing during the whole movement.

C1 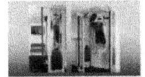 **Pull Up - Narrow Grip**
Sets: 2   Reps: 12-15
Tempo: Fast Intensity: 15RM

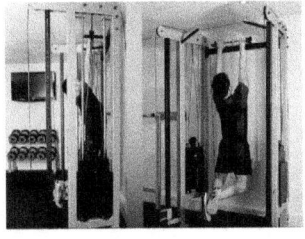 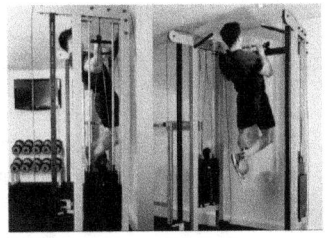

- Stand under the chin up bar at a height where you are able to grip the bar without jumping.

-Take hold of the bar with both hands facing away from you and inside shoulder width apart. Bring your shoulder blades back towards each other and down towards your bum.

- Pull yourself up to the top position. Your chin should be above your hands and chest pushed out.

- From the top position, lower your self down under control to the bottom.

C2 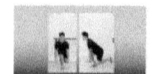 **Single Leg Dead Lift with Dumbbells**
Sets: 2   Reps: 12-15
Tempo: Fast Intensity: 15RM

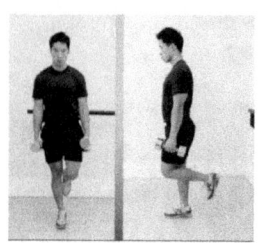 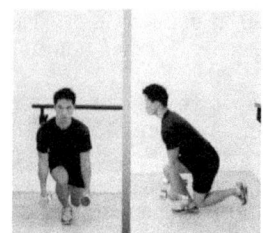

- Take a dumbbell in each hand.

- Stand on one leg with your hips, chest and head facing forward. Gently draw in your tummy with 30% effort.

- Push your chest out and hollow your lower back.

- Bend your standing knee and lean slightly forward to touch dumbbells to the ground in line with the toes of your standing leg.

- Push through your standing leg and straighten into an upright standing position.

- Keep your chest pushed out, back hollowed and your hips facing forward throughout the whole movement.

D1 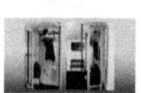 **Chin Up - Supinated Shoulder width Grip**
Sets: 2   Reps: 12-15
Tempo: Fast Intensity: 15RM

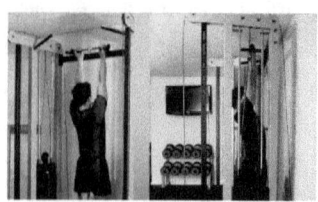 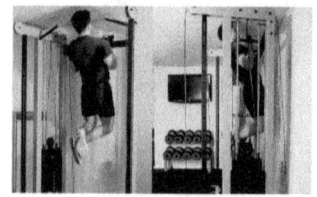

- Stand under the chin up bar at a height where you are able to grip the bar without jumping.

-Take hold of the bar with both hands facing you and shoulder width apart. Bring your shoulder blades back towards each other and down towards your bum.

- Pull yourself up to the top position. Your chin should be above your hands and chest pushed out.

- From the top position, lower your self down under control to the bottom.

D2 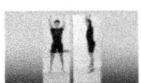 **Squat Jump**
Sets: 2   Reps: 12-15
Tempo: Fast Intensity: 15RM

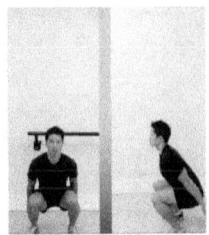 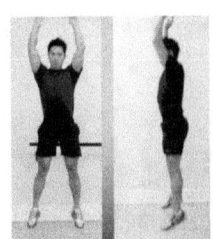

- Stand with your feet parallel and a comfortable distance apart with your weight evenly distributed between both legs.

- Keeping your chest up, bend at your knees then hips to lower your bum down towards the ground behind you.

- Go as low as you can with control, ideally your hips should go below your knees. Keeping your weight evenly distributed, jump up fast and as high as you can.

- When you land come down in to the bottom position before jumping up again.

E1 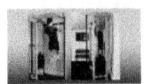 **Chin Up - Neutral Grip**
Sets: 2   Reps: 12-15
Tempo: Fast Intensity: 15RM

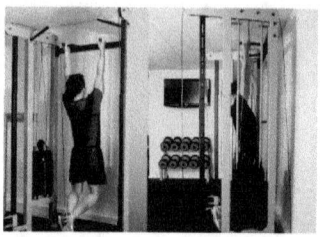 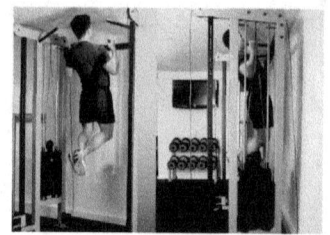

- Stand under the chin up bar at a height where you are able to grip the bar without jumping.

-Take hold of the bar with both hands facing each other. Bring your shoulder blades back towards each other and down towards your bum.

- Pull yourself up to the top position. Your chin should be above your hands and chest pushed out.

- From the top position, lower your self down under control to the bottom.

E2 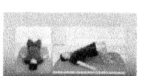 **Supine Bridge**
Sets: 2   Reps: 12-15
Tempo: Fast Intensity: 15RM

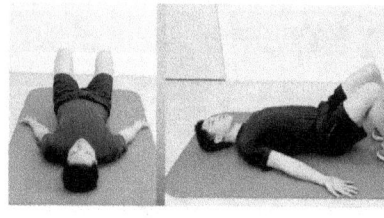 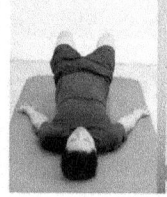 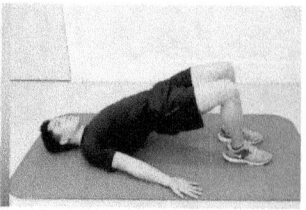

- Lie face up on a mat.

- Bend your knees so your feet are flat on the floor with heels under knees.

- Push through your heels, lifting your hips up to the point where there is a straight line from your chest to your knees. Squeeze your bum at the top of the movement.

- Lower until your bum is just above the ground and lift again.

- Keep your hips aligned throughout the whole movement.

Phase: Circuit 2 - Program 1

A1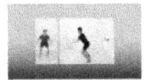
Bunny Hops
Sets: 2   Reps: 30sec
Tempo: Fast Rest: 30sec

B1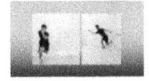
Ice Skaters
Sets: 2   Reps: 30sec
Tempo: Fast Rest: 30sec

C1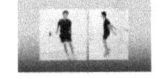
Metabolic Sideways Jumps
Sets: 2   Reps: 30sec
Tempo: Fast Rest: 30sec

D1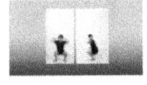
Prisoner Squat Jumps
Sets: 2   Reps: 30sec
Tempo: Fast Rest: 30sec

E1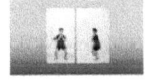
Plyometric Jump
Sets: 2   Reps: 30sec
Tempo: Fast Rest: 30sec

F1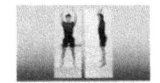
Squat Jump
Sets: 2   Reps: 30sec
Tempo: Fast Rest: 30sec

G1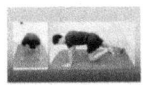
Press Up with Knee Tuck
Sets: 2   Reps: 30sec
Tempo: Fast Rest: 30sec

H1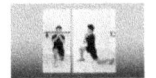
Squat, Jump Lunges
Sets: 2   Reps: 30sec
Tempo: Fast Rest: 30sec

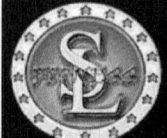
Phase: Circuit 2 - Program 1

A1 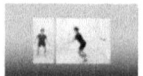 **Bunny Hops**
Sets: 2   Reps: 30sec
Tempo: Fast Rest: 30sec

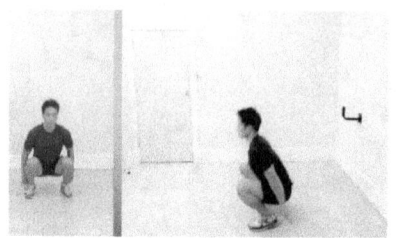 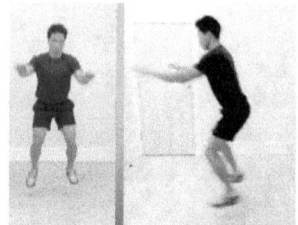

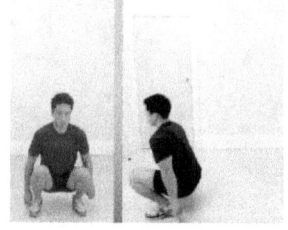

- Stand with your feet a comfortable distance apart.

- Bend at your knees then hips to lower your bum down towards the ground behind you. Start as low as you can with a slight forward lean.

- Spring forward and up as far as you can

- Land on both feet and repeat.

B1 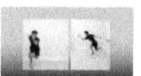 **Ice Skaters**
Sets: 2   Reps: 30sec
Tempo: Fast Rest: 30sec

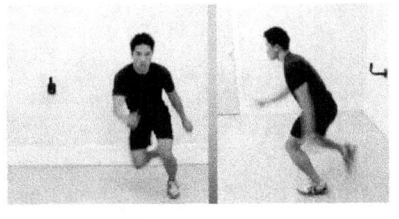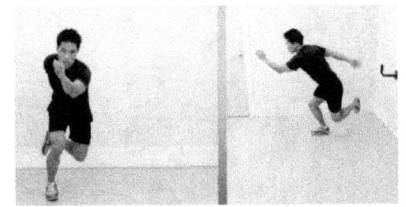

- Stand with your weight on one foot.

- Jump sideways as far as you can to land on the other foot.

- On landing jump again to land on the first foot.

- Look straight ahead throughout the movement.

C1 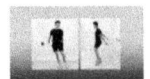 **Metabolic Sideways Jumps**
Sets: 2   Reps: 30sec
Tempo: Fast Rest: 30sec

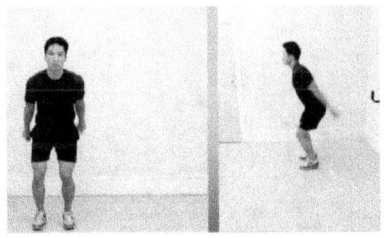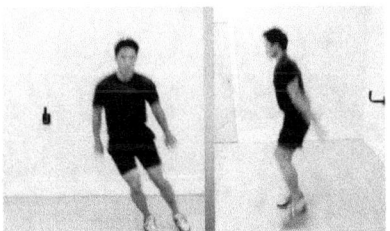

- Stand with your feet a comfortable distance apart

- Keeping your chest up, bend at your knees then hips quickly to lower your bum down towards the ground behind you.

- Spring sideways and up as far as you can.

- Land on both feet and repeat jumping back to the other side.

D1 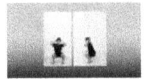 **Prisoner Squat Jumps**
Sets: 2   Reps: 30sec
Tempo: Fast Rest: 30sec

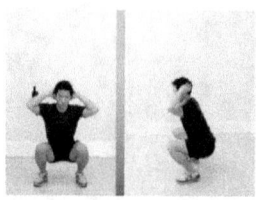 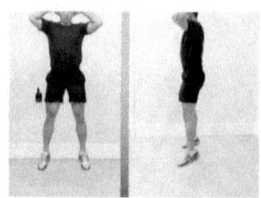

- Stand with your feet parallel and a comfortable distance apart with your weight evenly distributed between both legs.

- Put both hands up to the back or sides of your head, engage the muscles between your shoulder blades to bring your elbows high and wide . Make sure you don't put any pressure on your head pushing it forward.

- Keeping your chest up, bend at your knees then hips to lower your bum down towards the ground behind you.

- Go as low as you can with control, ideally your hips should go below your knees. Keeping your weight evenly distributed, jump up fast and as high as you can.

- When you land come down in to the bottom position before jumping up again.

E1 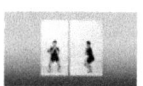 **Plyometric Jump**
Sets: 2   Reps: 30sec
Tempo: Fast Rest: 30sec

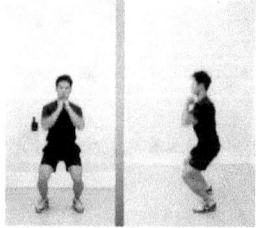 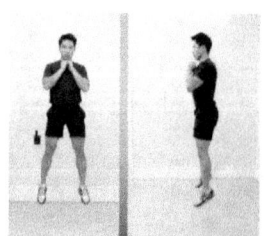

- Stand with your feet a comfortable distance apart.

- Keeping your chest up bend at your knees then hips to lower your bum down towards the ground behind you.

- Push up fast and jump as high as you can.

- Land on both feet and jump back up with as little contact time with the ground as possible.

F1 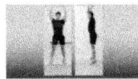 **Squat Jump**
Sets: 2   Reps: 30sec
Tempo: Fast Rest: 30sec

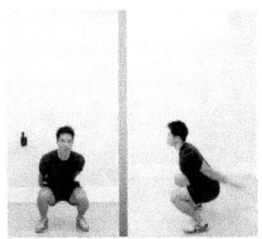 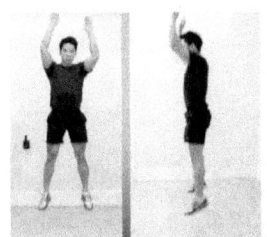

- Stand with your feet parallel and a comfortable distance apart with your weight evenly distributed between both legs.

- Keeping your chest up, bend at your knees then hips to lower your bum down towards the ground behind you.

- Go as low as you can with control, ideally your hips should go below your knees. Keeping your weight evenly distributed, jump up fast and as high as you can.

- When you land come down in to the bottom position before jumping up again.

G1 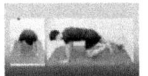 **Press Up with Knee Tuck**
Sets: 2   Reps: 30sec
Tempo: Fast Rest: 30sec

Sorry, no photos are available for this exercise

Press Up
- Come down so that your hands and feet are on the floor.

- Place your hands a little wider than shoulder width apart.

- Position your hips to form a straight line from your heels to your head.

- Gently draw in your tummy using roughly 30% effort.

- Bend your elbows lowering your body toward the ground. Keep your elbows at about 45 degrees from the sides of your body.

- You should come down so that your chest is between your hands.

- Lower until your chest is a small fist away from the ground and then push back up to the start position.

116

Knee Tuck
- In the top position bend one knee and bring it up towards your chest, then return the foot to its grounded position.

- Repeat on the other leg.

H1 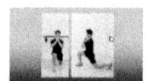 **Squat, Jump Lunges**
Sets: 2   Reps: 30sec
Tempo: Fast Rest: 30sec

Sorry, no photos are available for this exercise

Squat
- Stand with your feet parallel and a comfortable distance apart with your weight evenly distributed between both legs.

- Keeping your chest up, bend at your knees then hips to lower your bum down towards the ground behind you.

- Go as low as you can with control, ideally your hips should go below your knees. Keeping your heels on the ground, push up into the start position.

Jump Lunges
- Jump one leg forward and the other back to create a stride approximately 1 ½ times your natural stride length.

- Putting your weight on your front leg lower yourself forward and down.

- Coming down keep your back knee behind your hips. Your back heel should come off the ground.

- From the bottom position jump back and up and switch your legs around

- Once done on both legs jump back in to the starting squat position.

Phase: Circuit 2 - Program 2

A1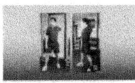
Static Pectoral Stretch with 90 Degree Bent Elbow
Sets: 1 Reps: 30 sec

A2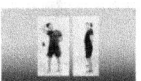
Upper Trap Stretch
Sets: 1 Reps: 30 sec

A3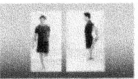
Standing Static Quadriceps Stretch
Sets: 1 Reps: 30 sec

A4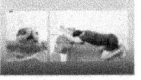
Static Lat Stretch, Elbows on Bench
Sets: 1 Reps: 30 sec

A5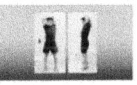
Triceps Overhead Stretch
Sets: 1 Reps: 30 sec

A6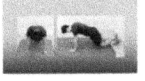
Prone Soleus Stretch
Sets: 1 Reps: 30 sec

A7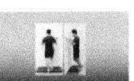
Single Leg Gastrocnemius Stretch from Step
Sets: 1 Reps: 30 sec

A8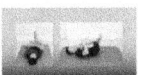
Lying Supine Glute Stretch
Sets: 1 Reps: 30 sec

A9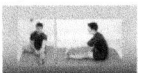
Seated Hamstring Stretch
Sets: 1 Reps: 30 sec ·

A10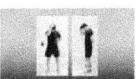
Occipital Stretch
Sets: 1 Reps: 30 sec

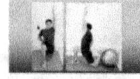
A11 **Kneeling Rectus Femoris Stretch**
Sets: 1 Reps: 30 sec

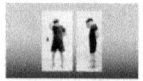
A12 **Levator Scapula Stretch**
Sets: 1 Reps: v30 sec

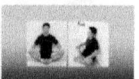
A13 **PNF Seated Adductor Stretch**
Sets: 1 Reps: 30 sec

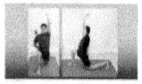
A14 **Kneeling Psoas Stretch**
Sets: 1 Reps: 30 sec

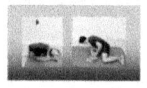
A15 **90/ 90 Glute Stretch**
Sets: 1 Reps: 30 sec

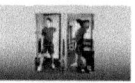
A16 **PNF Pectoral Stretch**
Sets: 1 Reps: 30 sec

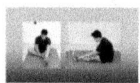
A17 **PNF Hamstring Stretch**
Sets: 1 Reps: 30 sec

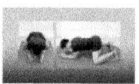
A18 **Adductor Stretch on Knees**
Sets: 1 Reps: 30 sec

Phase: Circuit 2 - Program 2

A1 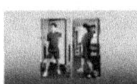 **Static Pectoral Stretch with 90 Degree Bent Elbow**
Sets: 1 Reps: 30 sec

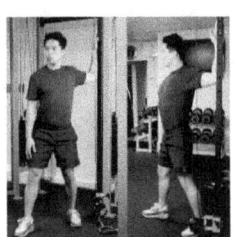

- Stand next to a doorway or corner of a wall. Put the palm and elbow of one arm on the wall with a 90 degree bend at the elbow. Your elbow should be slightly above your shoulder.

- Keeping your hand and elbow on the wall, turn away from that arm and stretch your chest.

A2 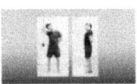 **Upper Trap Stretch**
Sets: 1 Reps: 30 sec

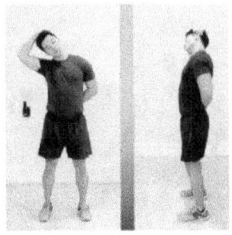

- Stand with your feet hip width apart.

- Bend one elbow and bring that arm behind your back.

- Lean your head over to the other side and use your free hand to add some pressure to the stretch.

A3 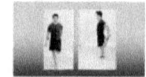 **Standing Static Quadriceps Stretch**
Sets: 1 Reps: 30 sec

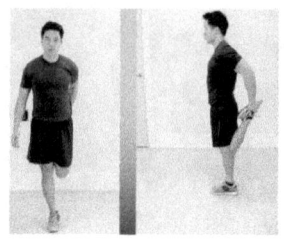

- Stand with your feet hip width apart.

- Bend at the knee of one leg. Use your corresponding hand to take hold of your ankle and pull it towards your bum.

- Squeeze your bum and gently push your hips forward to increase the stretch.

A4 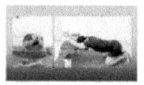 **Static Lat Stretch, Elbows on Bench**
Sets: 1 Reps: 30 sec

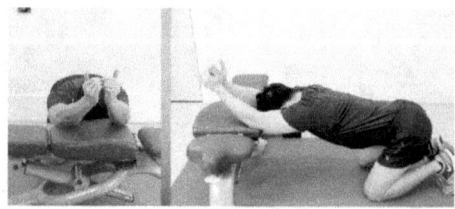

- Kneel on the floor with a bench in front of you.

- Lean over and put your elbows on the bench. Bend at your elbows.

- Push your chest out and keep your head in a neutral position then come down as low as you can to create a stretch down the sides of you back and behind your shoulders.

A5 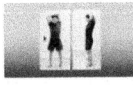 **Triceps Overhead Stretch**
Sets: 1 Reps: 30 sec

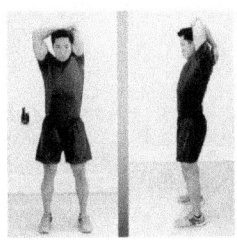

- Stand with your feet hip width apart.

- Bring one arm over your head and bend your elbow to put your palm on your back.

- Use your free hand to pull and add some pressure to the stretch.

A6 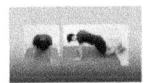 **Prone Soleus Stretch**
Sets: 1 Reps: 30 sec

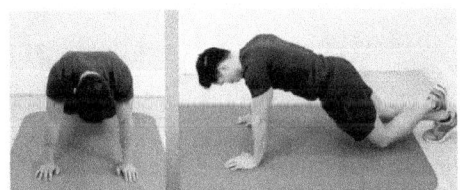

- Put your hands and feet on the ground while facing down.

- Straighten your knees and try to push one heel down towards the ground.

- Cross your other leg over the top to apply extra pressure to the stretch.

- Bend the knee of the leg you are stretching. You should feel the stretch move lower down your leg.

A7 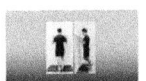 **Single Leg Gastrocnemius Stretch from Step**
Sets: 1 Reps: 30 sec

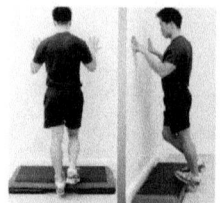

- Stand on a step put your hands on a wall or banister for support.

- Make sure the step is sturdy and will not flip over.

- Drop the heel of one foot down from the edge of the step with your weight on the ball of that foot.

- Take your other foot off the step so your full weight is going into the stretch.

A8 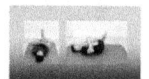 **Lying Supine Glute Stretch**
Sets: 1 Reps: 30 sec

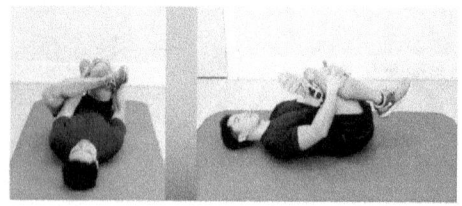

- Lie on your back with legs outstretched.

- Bend a knee then cross the ankle of your other leg in front of that knee.

- Use your hands to pull the knee and crossed over ankle up towards your body.

A9 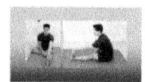 **Seated Hamstring Stretch**
Sets: 1 Reps: 30 sec

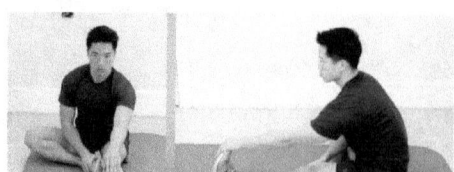

- Sit with one leg stretched out in front of your body and the other bent with your knee out to the side.

- Lean forward towards the foot of your stretched out leg and bring your hands as far down the leg as you can.

A10 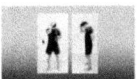 **Occipital Stretch**
Sets: 1 Reps: 30 sec

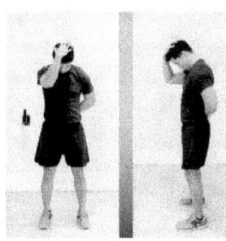

- Stand with your feet hip width apart.

- Bend one elbow and bring that arm behind your back.

- Lean your head forward. Use your free hand to add some pressure to the stretch.

A11 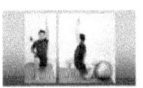 **Kneeling Rectus Femoris Stretch**
Sets: 1 Reps: 30 sec

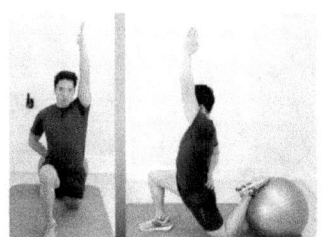

- Kneel on a mat with one leg and bring the other forward with knee bent and foot flat on the ground.

- Raise your back foot up towards your bum and support it on a swiss ball or step.

- Extend the arm corresponding with the kneeling leg over your head.

- Squeeze your bum and push your hips forward to feel a stretch in your kneeling leg.

A12 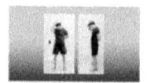 **Levator Scapula Stretch**
Sets: 1 Reps: v30 sec

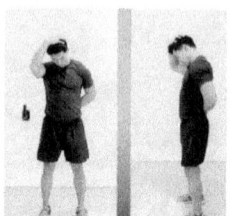

- Stand with your feet hip width apart.

- Bend one elbow and bring that arm behind your back.

- Lean your head forward and to the other side as if looking down at a jeans front pocket. Use your free hand to add some pressure to the stretch.

A13 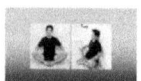 **PNF Seated Adductor Stretch**
Sets: 1 Reps: 30 sec

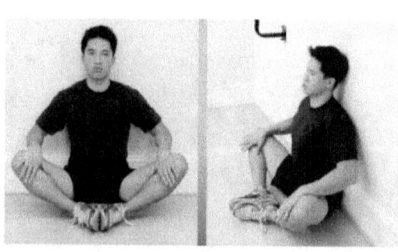 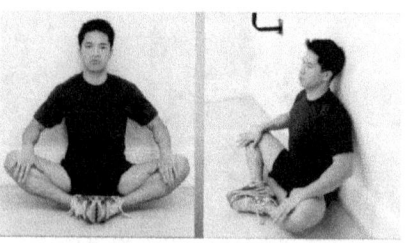

- Sit with your back against a wall. Bend and turn out your knees bringing the soles of your feet together.

- Bring your knees down towards the ground, use your hands to apply a gentle pressure. Hold for approximately 5 seconds.

-Then using your adductor muscles (groin) push your knees up in to your hands with about 30 percent effort. Hold this push for approximately 5 seconds.

- Relax your muscles and using your hands push your knees down again, this time a little further than before.

- Repeat this process multiple times slightly increasing the effort of your push up each time and slightly increasing the range of the stretch each time.

A14 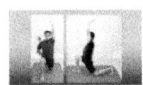 **Kneeling Psoas Stretch**
Sets: 1 Reps: 30 sec

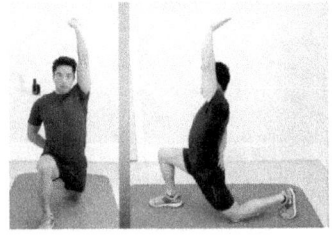

- Kneel on a mat with one leg and bring the other forward with knee bent and foot flat on the ground. Your back toes should be tucked under your heel.

- Extend the arm corresponding with the kneeling leg over your head. Have your palm facing up.

- Squeeze your bum and push your hips forward to feel a stretch at the top of your kneeling leg.

A15 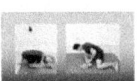 **90/ 90 Glute Stretch**
Sets: 1 Reps: 30 sec

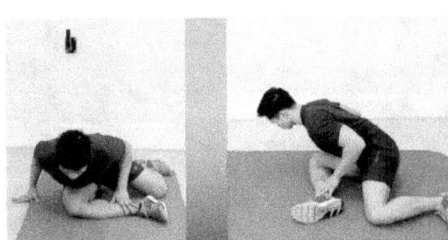 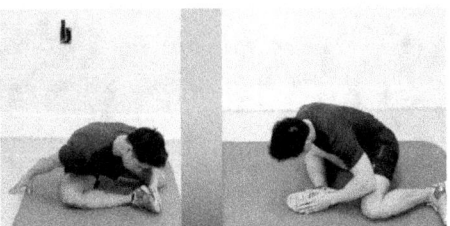

- Sit with one leg out in front of your hips and one leg behind. Bend both knees to 90 degrees.

- Lean forward towards your front knee to feel a stretch in your bum and lower back.

- Lift your torso up to release the stretch.

- Repeat the movement using your outside arm to push your torso in towards your front foot. You should feel a stretch in the bum, lower back and outside of your front leg.

A16 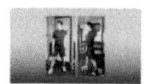 **PNF Pectoral Stretch**
Sets: 1 Reps: 30 sec

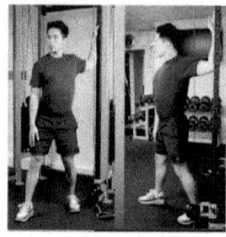

- Stand next to a doorway or corner of a wall. Put the palm and elbow of one arm on the wall with a 90 degree bend at the elbow. Your elbow should be slightly above your shoulder.

- Keeping your hand and elbow on the wall, turn away from that arm and stretch your chest. Hold for approximately 5 seconds.

-Then using your pectoral (chest) muscles push in to the wall with about 30 percent effort. Hold this push for approximately 5 seconds.

- Relax your muscles and turn away again to stretch your chest, this time a little further than before.

- Repeat this process multiple times slightly increasing the effort of your push each time and slightly increasing the range of the stretch each time.

A17 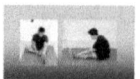 **PNF Hamstring Stretch**
Sets: 1 Reps: 30 sec

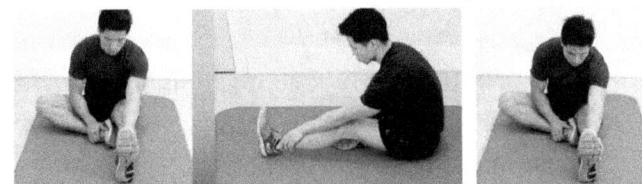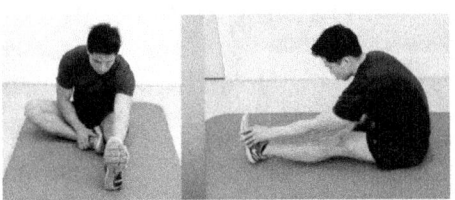

- Sit with one leg stretched out in front of your body and the other bent with your knee out to the side.

- Lean forward towards the foot of your stretched out leg and bring your hands as far down the leg as you can. Hold for approximately 5 seconds.

-Then bend at your knee and push your heel in to the ground and towards your bum to contract your hamstring muscles with about 30 percent effort. Hold this contraction for approximately 5 seconds.

- Relax your muscles, straighten your leg and lean forward to stretch once again, this time a little further than before.

- Repeat this process multiple times slightly increasing the effort of your contraction each time and slightly increasing the range of the stretch each time.

A18 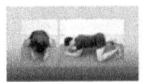 **Adductor Stretch on Knees**
Sets: 1 Reps: 30 sec

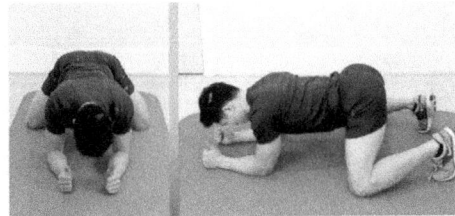

- Come down on to both knees. Push your chest out and bring your shoulders back.

- Widen your knees to bring a slight stretch to the inside of your legs.

- Keeping your chest out and shoulders back, lean forward from your hips to bring your hands and then elbows towards the floor.

- Bring your knees a little wider to get a good stretch.

Walking & Running Programs

Included here are some sample walking programs. There are a walk and a run walk program to get you ready to run your first 5k. These are an excellent way to begin a cardiovascular program and see if running is something you enjoy. On our website, we offer other running programs that you can purchase to help you progress and achieve better race results.

5k Walk Program

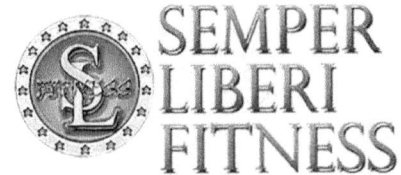

5k Walk Program – This is a basic beginner program designed to help promote physical activity. It was designed to be the first step in a more active lifestyle that anyone at any physical ability level could use to begin their path to a more active lifestyle.

There are three scheduled walking days with two Walk/Activity days to promote activity. Do not let these added days intimidate you if you are a beginner. These extra two days allow for multiple extra activities such as Strength Training, Athletics, Martial Arts, or even just playing active games with family & friends. They can be anything to help maintain a more active lifestyle. If you are having any problems with recovery, utilize these days for extra rest. This should not be needed for most participants due to the low intensity of the beginner program.

The program includes the volume progression graph showing the intended increases in volume to allow for adaptation. These graphs will show a visual representation of workload and the tapering before the final 5k event.

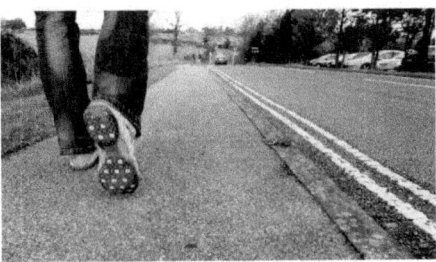

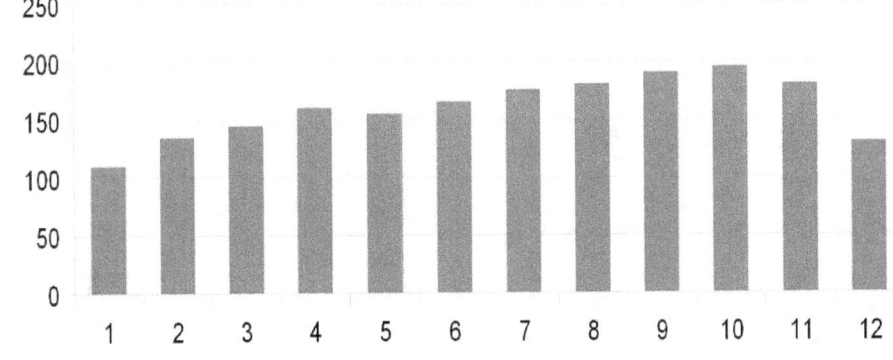

Stretching

- Stretching helps increase flexibility and can help alleviate soreness and aid recovery. You can stretch for a few minutes after warm-up if you feel it is needed (never stretch a cold muscle) but ensure you stretch after exercise as it will help with recovery.
- Here are a few recommendations for stretching for more resources view our website flexibility section.
- Hold each stretch for 30 to 40 seconds. Do not stretch until discomfort, only until you feel a stretch in the muscle and then hold that position for the
- 30-40 sec. If you have problems with a particular area, stretch that area twice. (hold for 30-40 seconds release, and then stretch again.)
- **Calf Stretch** – Find a step or curb near a railing, Use the railing for balance and let your heels hang off the edge of the surface. Allow you heels to drop stretching you calf and Achilles tendon. Hold this position. Be sure to keep your body upright and straight. Release and repeat. You can do this with a single leg or both whichever make you more comfortable. Always try to work to unilateral (one-sided) moves in all stretching to help improve balance and coordination.
- **Hamstring Stretch**
- **Standing** – Stand in a shoulder width stance with the load bearing (non-stretching) foot facing forward and the non-load bearing stretching foot at a 45-degree angle. Slightly bend the load bearing leg's knee while keeping the stretching leg straight and picking the toes of the stretching leg off the ground. Begin to bend over while reaching toward the toes of the stretching leg. Continue to shift weight to load bearing leg and increasing the bend in the knee until you feel a stretch in the desired leg. Repeat with the other leg.
- **Seated** - While sitting at the edge of a chair, straighten one leg in front of the body with the heel on the floor. Then, sit up straight and try pushing the navel towards the thigh without leaning the trunk of the body forwards. If you are flexible enough that this version does not give you a sufficient stretch prop your feet on a stool or chair and follow the same steps. The added elevation of the stretching leg should allow for a greater stretch in the hamstring.

Standing Quadriceps Stretch   **Standing Calf Stretch**

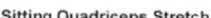

Sitting Quadriceps Stretch

Standing Hamstring Stretch

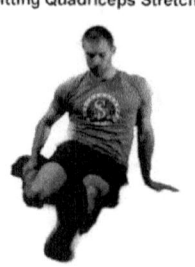

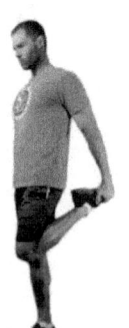

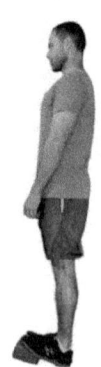

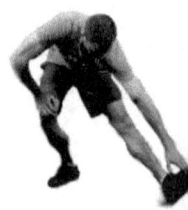

⭐ SEMPER LIBERI
Endurance Program

Day	Sun.	Mon.	Tues.	Wed.	Thur.	Fri.	Sat.
Mode	Off	Walk	Walk or Activity	Speed Walk Intervals	Off	Walk or Activity	Walk
Intensity	Off	Low	Medium	High/Low	Off	Medium	Med./High
HR	Off	55-65%	55-65%	65-80%	Off	65-75%	70-80%
RPE	Off	5-6	6-7	7+	Off	6-7	7+
Week 1	Off	20 Min.	25 Min.	20 Min.	Off	20 Min.	25 Min.
Week 2	Off	25 Min.	30 Min.	25 Min.	Off	25 Min.	30 Min.
Week 3	Off	30 Min.	25 Min.	25 Min.	Off	30 Min.	35 Min.
Week 4	Off	30 Min.	30 Min.	30 Min.	Off	30 Min.	40 Min.
Week 5	Off	30 Min.	30 Min.	30 Min.	Off	30 Min.	35 Min.
Week 6	Off	30 Min.	30 Min.	35 Min.	Off	30 Min.	40 Min.
Week 7	Off	35 Min.	30 Min.	35 Min.	Off	30 Min.	45 Min.
Week 8	Off	35 Min.	30 Min.	35 Min.	Off	30 Min.	50 Min.
Week 9	Off	35 Min.	20 Min.	40 Min.	Off	30 Min.	55 Min.
Week 10	Off	35 Min.	30 Min.	40 Min.	Off	20 Min.	60 Min.
Week 11	Off	35 Min.	30 Min.	40 Min.	Off	20 Min.	45 Min.
Week 12	Off	20 Min.	30 Min.	35 Min.	Off	30 Min.	5K Walk

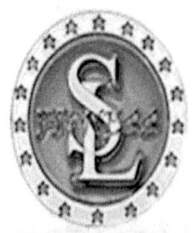 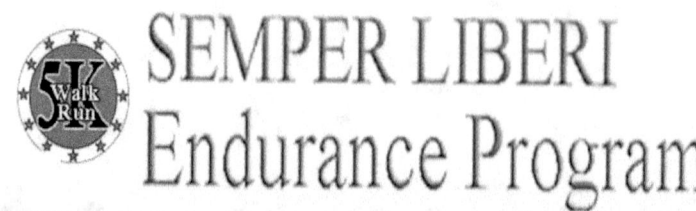

SEMPER LIBERI
Endurance Program

Day	Sun.	Mon.	Tues.	Wed.	Thur.	Fri.	Sat.
Mode	Off	Walk/Run	Walk or Activity	Walk/Run	Off	Walk or Activity	Walk/Run
Intensity	Off	Med./High	Medium	Med./High	Off	Medium	Medium
HR	Off	65-80%	65-75%	65-80%	Off	65-75%	65-75%
RPE	Off	6-7+	6-7	6-7+	Off	6-7	6-7
Week 1	Off	3 Min. Walk/1 Min. Run For 20 Min.	30 Min.	3 Min Walk/1 Min. Run For 20 Min.	Off	30 Min.	3 Min Walk/1 Min. Run For 24 Min.
Week 2	Off	1 Min. Walk/3 Min. Run For 24 Min.	30 Min.	1 Min. Walk/3 Min. Run For 24 Min.	Off	30 Min.	2 Min. Walk/2 Min. Run For 30 Min.
Week 3	Off	2 Min. Walk/2 Min. Run For 30 Min.	30 Min.	1 Min. Walk/3 Min. Run For 24 Min.	Off	30 Min.	2 Min. Walk/2 Min. Run For 36 Min.
Week 4	Off	1 Min. Walk/3 Min. Run For 30 Min.	30 Min.	1 Min. Walk/3 Min. Run For 30 Min.	Off	30 Min.	2 Min. Walk/2 Min. Run For 40 Min.
Week 5	Off	2 Min. Walk/2 Min. Run For 30 Min.	30 Min.	1 Min. Walk/1 Min. Run For 30 Min.	Off	30 Min.	2 Min. Walk/2 Min. Run For 36 Min.
Week 6	Off	2 Min. Walk/2 Min. Run For 30 Min.	30 Min.	2 Min. Walk/2 Min. Run For 36 Min.	Off	30 Min.	2 Min. Walk/2 Min. Run For 40 Min.
Week 7	Off	2 Min. Walk/2 Min. Run For 34 Min.	30 Min.	2 Min. Walk/2 Min. Run For 36 Min.	Off	30 Min.	1 Min. Walk/3 Min. Run For 44 Min.
Week 8	Off	2 Min. Walk/2 Min. Run For 34 Min.	30 Min.	1 Min. Walk/3 Min. Run For 36 Min.	Off	30 Min.	2 Min. Walk/2 Min. Run For 50 Min.
Week 9	Off	2 Min. Walk/2 Min. Run For 34 Min.	20 Min.	2 Min. Walk/2 Min. Run For 40 Min.	Off	30 Min.	2 Min. Walk/2 Min. Run For 56 Min.
Week 10	Off	2 Min. Walk/2 Min. Run For 34 Min.	30 Min.	2 Min. Walk/2 Min. Run For 40 Min.	Off	30 Min.	2 Min. Walk/2 Min. Run For 60 Min.
Week 11	Off	1 Min. Walk/3 Min. Run For 34 Min.	30 Min.	2 Min. Walk/2 Min. Run For 40 Min.	Off	30 Min.	2 Min. Walk/2 Min. Run For 44 Min.
Week 12	Off	1 Min. Walk/3 Min. Run For 34 Min.	30 Min.	2 Min. Walk/2 Min. Run For 34 Min.	Off	30 Min.	5K

Cool Down - At the end of your walk you need to slow the pace to cool down. The harder you have worked out the longer you should cool down. In the beginning, your walks are very short, and you only need to cool down a couple of minutes. As your walking time and intensity extends so should your cool down period. After cool down stretch to help reduce Delayed Onset Muscle Soreness and increase flexibility to improve future performance.

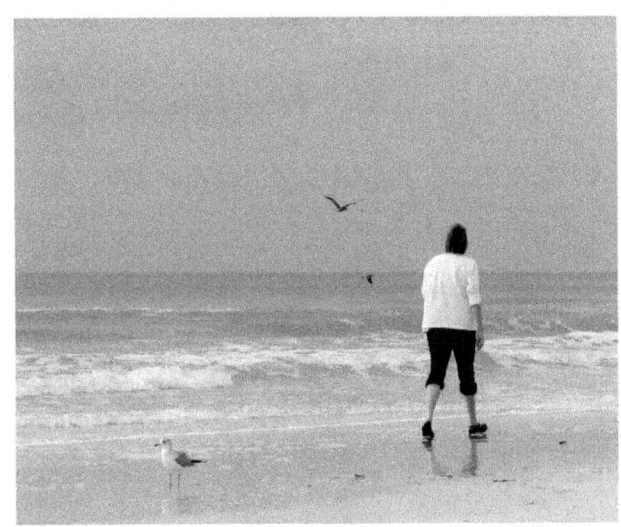

- **RPE (Rating of Perceived Exertion)** – is how hard your training feels to you. On a 1-10 scale how hard do you feel the exercise is at that point in time. RPE is a very individualized measurement as the exertion and effort one person may feel is going to be different from another. It will also vary from workout to workout and exercise to exercise. In interval training, the RPE may be an 8-9 on sprints and reduce to a 2-3 for recovery before sprinting again. RPE is an excellent tool to help beginners ensure they are not over training and thus prohibiting adequate recovery.

- **HR (Heart Rate)** – Heart rate is the most commonly used way to prescribe endurance activity due to the relationship between heart rate and oxygen consumption. Using the heart rate as a measurement will allow the program to be more specific to the individual and improve progress. Highly effective endurance programs require knowledge of energy systems and oxygen consumption in order to manage training intensity to improve endurance. In order to measure heart rate to ensure training in optimal exercise intensities a heart rate monitor is needed. The Sketchers Go Walk SK1 is a very easy to use and affordable option to track heart rate and other fitness and exercise goals.

- **Intervals** – Perform intervals at a 1-1 ratio with 1-min. at a slightly higher RPE or HR and then 1 min. at a slower recovery pace to rest. See Chart for RPE & HR protocols.

5k Walk/Run Program

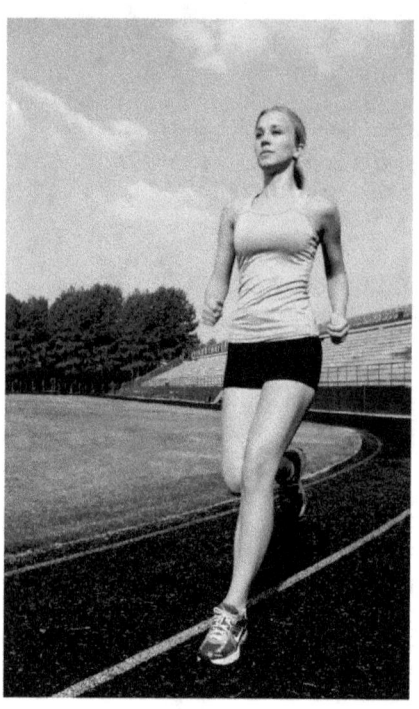

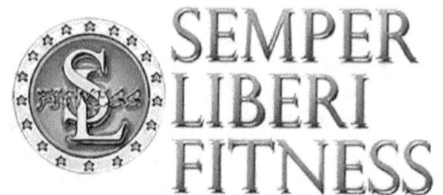

SEMPER LIBERI FITNESS

This program is the second step in the 5k journey. The program is similar to the regular walking program with three walking days and two activity days. Once again the activity days can be any activity as the main purpose of the programs is simply to promote activity. If you are having any problems with recovery, utilize these days for extra rest. This should not be needed for most participants due to the low intensity of the beginner program.

The major difference between this program and the walking program is the added intensity boosting days where you will run short intervals in order to increase running capacity. If you follow the suggested intensities and progress to the end of the program you will be on your way to continuously running for you workouts instead of walking.

The program includes the volume progression graph showing the intended increases in volume to allow for adaptation. These graphs will show a visual representation of workload and the tapering before the final 5k event.

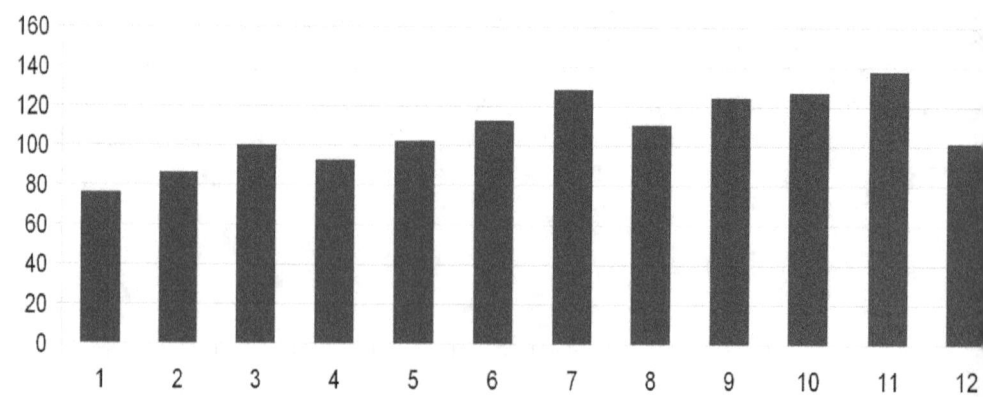

Stretching

• Stretching helps increase flexibility and can help alleviate soreness and aid recovery. You can stretch for a few minutes after warm-up if you feel it is needed (never stretch a cold muscle) but ensure you stretch after exercise as it will help with recovery.

• Here are a few recommendations for stretching for more resources view our website flexibility section.

• Hold each stretch for 30 to 40 seconds. Do not stretch until discomfort, only until you feel a stretch in the muscle and then hold that position for the

• 30-40 sec. If you have problems with a particular area, stretch that area twice. (hold for 30-40 seconds release, and then stretch again.)

• **Calf Stretch** – Find a step or curb near a railing, Use the railing for balance and let your heels hang off the edge of the surface. Allow you heels to drop stretching you calf and Achilles tendon. Hold this position. Be sure to keep your body upright and straight. Release and repeat. You can do this with a single leg or both whichever make you more comfortable. Always try to work to unilateral (one-sided) moves in all stretching to help improve balance and coordination.

• **Hamstring Stretch**

• **Standing** – Stand in a shoulder width stance with the load bearing (non-stretching) foot facing forward and the non-load bearing stretching foot at a 45-degree angle. Slightly bend the load bearing leg's knee while keeping the stretching leg straight and picking the toes of the stretching leg off the ground. Begin to bend over while reaching toward the toes of the stretching leg. Continue to shift weight to load bearing leg and increasing the bend in the knee until you feel a stretch in the desired leg. Repeat with the other leg.

• **Seated** - While sitting at the edge of a chair, straighten one leg in front of the body with the heel on the floor. Then, sit up straight and try pushing the navel towards the thigh without leaning the trunk of the body forwards. If you are flexible enough that this version does not give you a sufficient stretch prop your feet on a stool or chair and follow the same steps. The added elevation of the stretching leg should allow for a greater stretch in the hamstring.

Warm-Up – 5 min. of exercise at a lower intensity to get the blood circulating and let your body know that you are preparing for exercise. Warming up can be anything to get loose and ready for exercise. For many of your walks, it will only be necessary to warm up about five minutes usually by walking at a lower intensity than the prescribed daily plan. The more advanced you become, the more advanced the warm-up will need to be. For many of your walks, it will only be necessary to warm up about five minutes usually by walking at a lower intensity than the prescribed daily plan. As you progress through your walking program, you will need to warm up longer especially on days that you will do faster workouts.

Standing Quadriceps Stretch   Standing Calf Stretch

ng Quadriceps Stretch

Standing Hamstring Stretch

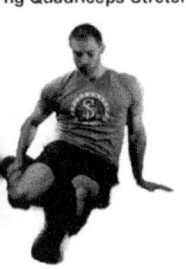
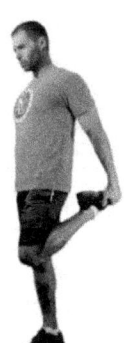
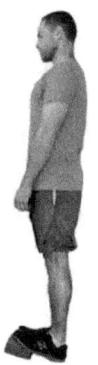
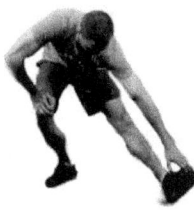

- **Cool Down** - At the end of your walk you need to slow the pace to cool down. The harder you have worked out the longer you should cool down. In the beginning, your walks are very short, and you only need to cool down a couple of minutes. As your walking time and intensity extends so should your cool down period. After cool down stretch to help reduce Delayed Onset Muscle Soreness and increase flexibility to improve future performance.

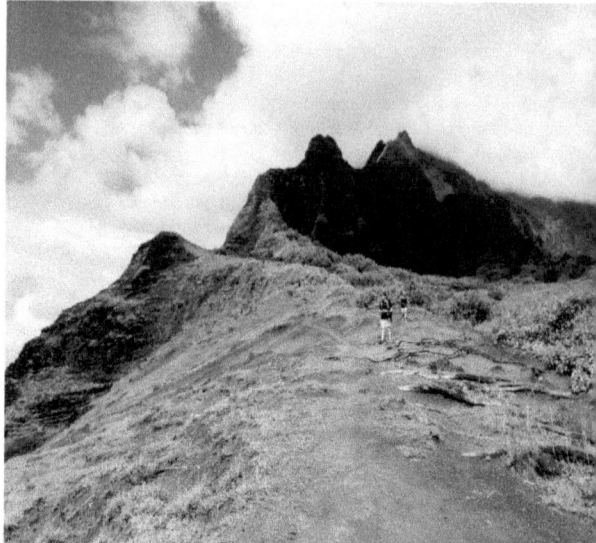

- **RPE (Rating of Perceived Exertion)** – is how hard your training feels to you. On a 1-10 scale how hard do you feel the exercise is at that point in time. RPE is a very individualized measurement as the exertion and effort one person may feel is going to be different from another. It will also vary from workout to workout and exercise to exercise. In interval training, the RPE may be an 8-9 on sprints and reduce to a 2-3 for recovery before sprinting again. RPE is an excellent tool to help beginners ensure they are not over training and thus prohibiting adequate recovery.

- **HR (Heart Rate)** – Heart rate is the most commonly used way to prescribe endurance activity due to the relationship between heart rate and oxygen consumption. Using the heart rate as a measurement will allow the program to be more specific to the individual and improve progress. Highly effective endurance programs require knowledge of energy systems and oxygen consumption in order to manage training intensity to improve endurance. In order to measure heart rate to ensure training in optimal exercise intensities a heart rate monitor is needed. The Sketchers Go Walk SK1 is a very easy to use and affordable option to track heart rate and other fitness and exercise goals.

- **Intervals** – Perform intervals at a 1-1 ratio with 1-min. at a slightly higher RPE or HR and then 1 min. at a slower recovery pace to rest. See Chart for RPE & HR protocols.

Martial Arts

I wanted to include a small program to give you an idea of what Karate and Krav Maga entail. I am not certified or a professional in martial arts. I have several years of experience and have coached white belt beginners so I do have an idea of what a good program requires. However, I wanted to make these cardiovascular in nature so they are structured more as a fitness program than a martial arts program. These are martial arts moves, but they are structured to help burn fat. If you enjoy the movements be sure to contact a local dojo and inquire further so you can get the real martial arts experience.

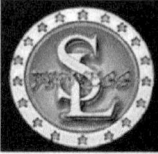

Phase: Martial Arts

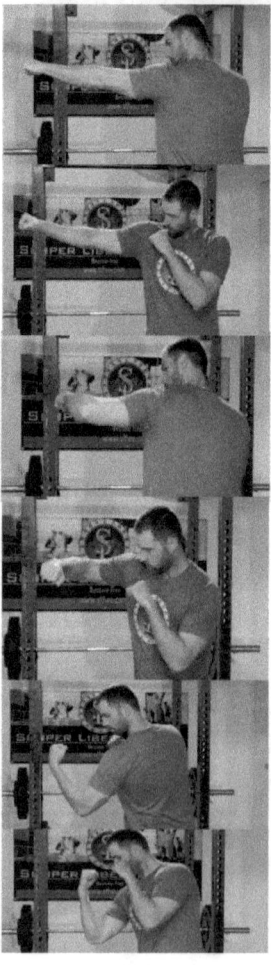

Jabs Left
Sets - 1 Reps - 20 Rest - None

Jabs Right
Sets - 1 Reps - 20 Rest - None

Hook Left
Sets - 1 Reps - 20 Rest - None

Hook Right
Sets - 1 Reps - 20 Rest - None

Uppercut Left
Sets - 1 Reps - 20 Rest - None

Uppercut Right
Sets - 1 Reps - 20 Rest - None

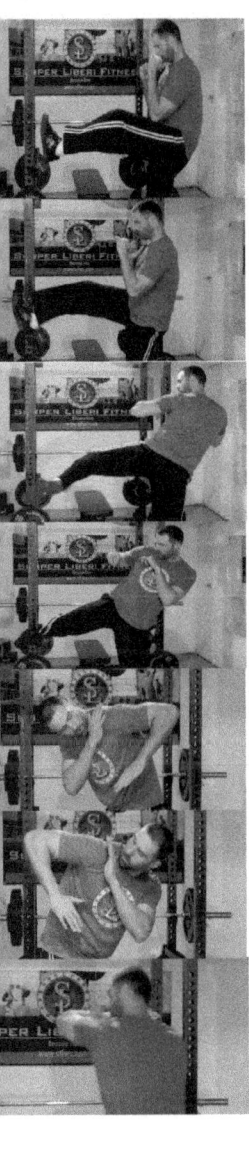

Straight Kick Left
Sets - 1 Reps - 20 Rest - None

Straight Kick Right
Sets - 1 Reps - 20 Rest - None

Round Kick Left
Sets - 1 Reps - 20 Rest - None

Round Kick Right
Sets - 1 Reps - 20 Rest - None

Upward Elbow Left
Sets - 1 Reps - 20 Rest - None

Upward Elbow Right
Sets - 1 Reps - 20 Rest - None

Cross Elbow Left
Sets - 1 Reps - 20 Rest - None

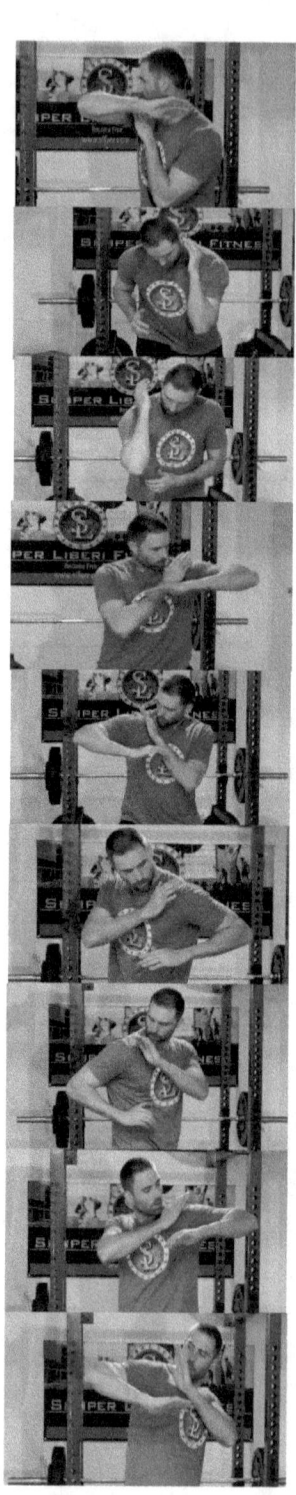

Cross Elbow Right
Sets - 1 Reps - 20 Rest - None

Downward Elbow Left
Sets - 1 Reps - 20 Rest - None

Downward Elbow Right
Sets - 1 Reps - 20 Rest - None

Side Elbow Left
Sets - 1 Reps - 20 Rest - None

Side Elbow Right
Sets - 1 Reps - 20 Rest - None

Back Elbow Left
Sets - 1 Reps - 20 Rest - None

Back Elbow Right
Sets - 1 Reps - 20 Rest - None

High Back Elbow Left
Sets - 1 Reps - 20 Rest - None

High Back Elbow Right
Sets - 1 Reps - 20 Rest - None

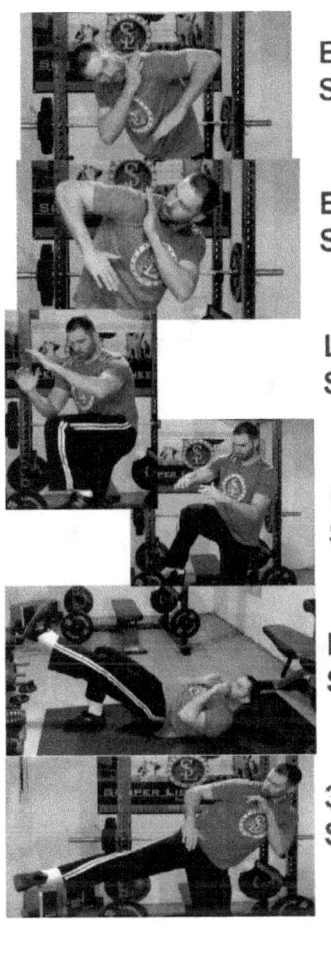

Back Uppward Elbow Left
Sets - 1 Reps - 20 Rest - None

Back Upward Elbow Right
Sets - 1 Reps - 20 Rest - None

Left Knees
Sets - 1 Reps - 20 Rest - None

Right Knees
Sets - 1 Reps - 20 Rest - None

Lying Kicks Each Leg
Sets - 1 Reps - 20 Rest - None

30 Seconds of Freestyle
Sets - 1 Reps - 20 Rest - None

MetCons

These workouts are structured with similar training principles as Crossfit. They are designed with metabolic conditioning in mind and with the goal of training certain energy systems. Some of these same principles are used in running and many other fitness programs. If you enjoy these fast-paced programs, then I suggest you research your local Crossfit affiliates and begin taking classes. You cannot get the real Crossfit experience by using the site and training at home. It is really designed to be a social fitness experience with group classes and being in a group. If you are an extrovert, you will love it!

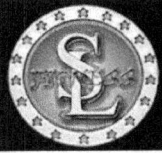

Phase: Met Con - Program 1

A1 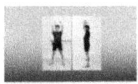 **Squat with Shoulder Press**
Sets: 1   Reps: 21
Tempo: Fast Rest: AsNec.

A2 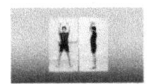 **Squat with Shoulder Press**
Sets: 1   Reps: 15
Tempo: Fast Rest: AsNec

A3 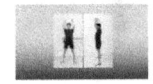 **Squat with Shoulder Press**
Sets: 1   Reps: 9
Tempo: Fast Rest: AsNec

B1 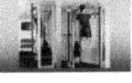 **Pull Up - Wide Grip**
Sets: 1   Reps: 21
Tempo: Fast Rest: AsNec

B2 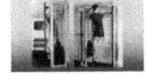 **Pull Up - Wide Grip**
Sets: 1   Reps: 15
Tempo: Fast Rest: AsNec

B3 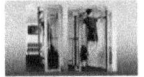 **Pull Up - Wide Grip**
Sets: 1   Reps: 9
Tempo: Fast Rest: AsNec

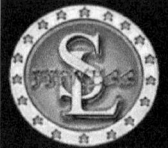
Phase: Met Con - Program 1

A1 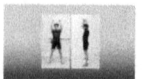 **Squat with Shoulder Press**
Sets: 1   Reps: 21
Tempo: Fast Rest: AsNec.

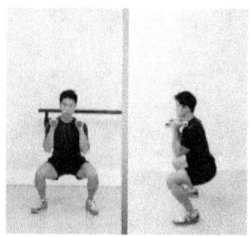 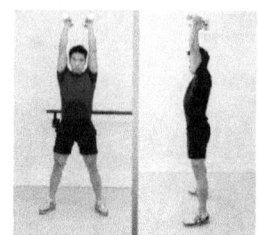

- Stand with your feet a comfortable distance apart. Take a dumbbell in each hand and hold them at shoulder height.

- Keeping your chest up, bend at your knees then hips to lower your bum down towards the ground behind you.

- Go as low as you can with control, ideally your hips should go below your knees.

- Keeping your heels on the ground, push up into the start position. Use the upward momentum to help you press the dumbbells up overhead directly above your shoulders.

- Bring the dumbbells back to the shoulder height position ready to go again.

A2 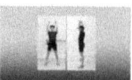 **Squat with Shoulder Press**
Sets: 1   Reps: 15
Tempo: Fast Rest: AsNec

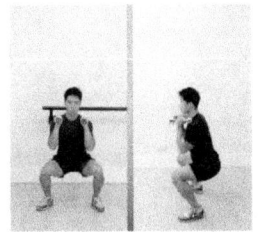 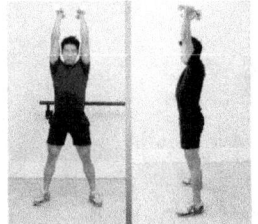

- Stand with your feet a comfortable distance apart. Take a dumbbell in each hand and hold them at shoulder height.

- Keeping your chest up, bend at your knees then hips to lower your bum down towards the ground behind you.

- Go as low as you can with control, ideally your hips should go below your knees.

- Keeping your heels on the ground, push up into the start position. Use the upward momentum to help you press the dumbbells up overhead directly above your shoulders.

- Bring the dumbbells back to the shoulder height position ready to go again.

A3 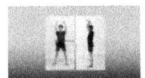 **Squat with Shoulder Press**
Sets: 1   Reps: 9
Tempo: Fast Rest: AsNec

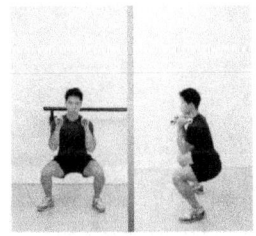 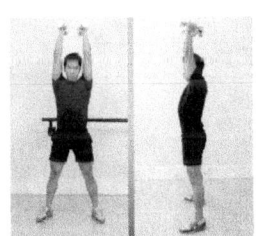

- Stand with your feet a comfortable distance apart. Take a dumbbell in each hand and hold them at shoulder height.

- Keeping your chest up, bend at your knees then hips to lower your bum down towards the ground behind you.

- Go as low as you can with control, ideally your hips should go below your knees.

- Keeping your heels on the ground, push up into the start position. Use the upward momentum to help you press the dumbbells up overhead directly above your shoulders.

- Bring the dumbbells back to the shoulder height position ready to go again.

B1 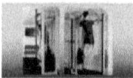 **Pull Up - Wide Grip**
Sets: 1   Reps: 21
Tempo: Fast Rest: AsNec

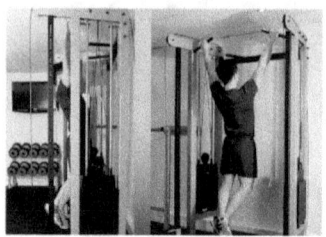 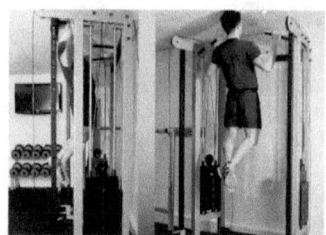

- Stand under the chin up bar at a height where you are able to grip the bar without jumping.

-Take hold of the bar with both hands facing away from you and 1 ½ times shoulder width apart. Bring your shoulder blades back towards each other and down towards your bum.

- Pull yourself up to the top position. Your chin should be above your hands and chest pushed out.

- From the top position, lower your self down under control to the bottom.

B2 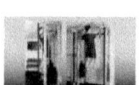 **Pull Up - Wide Grip**
Sets: 1   Reps: 15
Tempo: Fast Rest: AsNec

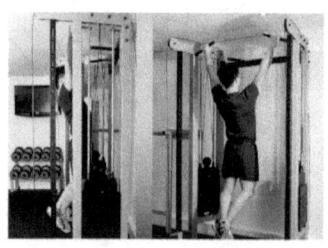 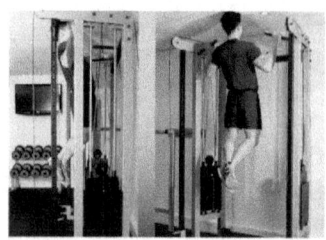

- Stand under the chin up bar at a height where you are able to grip the bar without

jumping.

-Take hold of the bar with both hands facing away from you and 1 ½ times shoulder width apart. Bring your shoulder blades back towards each other and down towards

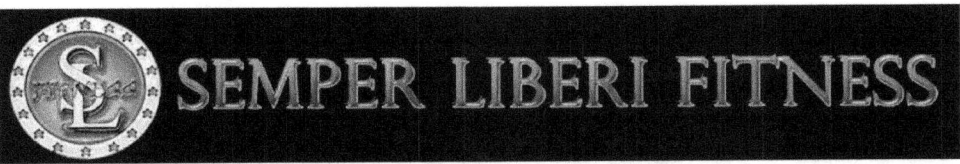

Phase: Met Con - Program 2

A1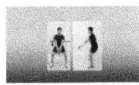

2 Arm Single Kettlebell Swing
Sets: 7   Reps: 15
Tempo: Fast Rest: AsNec

A2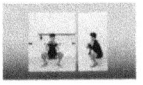

Clean
Sets: 7   Reps: 15
Tempo: Fast Rest: AsNec

A3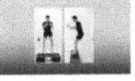

Box Jump
Sets: 7   Reps: 15
Tempo: Fast Rest: AsNec

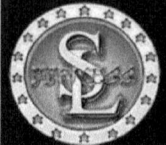

SEMPER LIBERI FITNESS

Phase: Met Con - Program 2

A1 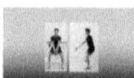 **2 Arm Single Kettlebell Swing**
Sets: 7   Reps: 15
Tempo: Fast Rest: AsNec

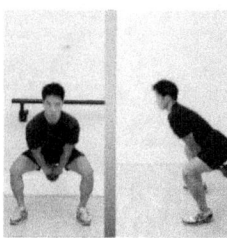 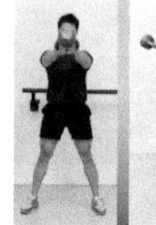 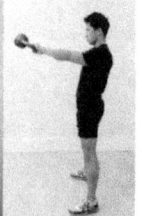

- Stand with your feet wider than shoulder width apart. Take a kettlebell in both hands, lean from your hips to put it on the ground a short distance in front of your body. Push your chest out to straighten your back.

- Keeping your back straight, lift the bell off the ground and swing it gently back between your legs. From this position thrust your hips forward and fully extend your body to power the bell out in front of your body.

- At shoulder height pull the kettlebell back down between your legs ready to thrust forward again.

- Your arms should remain extended throughout the movement.

- To end the movement just take the momentum out of the swing until the kettlebell stops in the bottom position and lower down to the floor.

A2 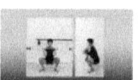 **Clean**
Sets: 7   Reps: 15
Tempo: Fast Rest: AsNec

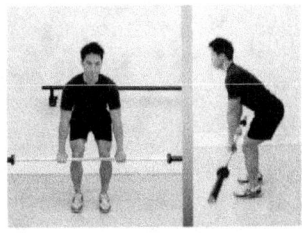 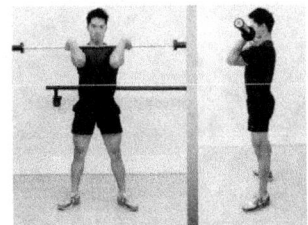

Stand with your feet parallel and shoulder width apart, with weight evenly distributed between both legs and the bar against your shins.

Grip the bar with both hands slightly wider than your legs, using a pronated grip.

Sink your bottom down towards the floor and with a straight back lift the bar up, keeping it against your shins.

As you approach your knees, take them back to allow the bar to clear them, and once cleared, bend the knees under the bar again.

As the bar reaches your upper legs, hit the bar off the top of your thighs, making it travel forward slightly. At this point you need to get under the bar in a wide front squat position, with the bar resting across the front of your shoulders and your elbows high.

Stand upright with the bar to finish the exercise.

A3 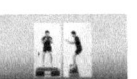 **Box Jump**
Sets: 7   Reps: 16
Tempo: Fast Rest: AsNec

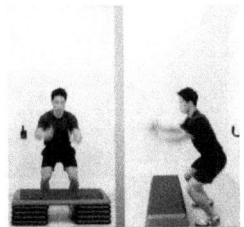 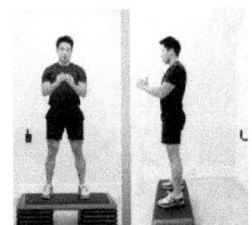

- Stand with your feet a comfortable distance apart with a step just in front of you.

- Keeping your chest up, bend at your knees then hips to lower your bum down towards the ground behind you.

- Push up fast and jump as high as you can.

- Land with both feet on the step.

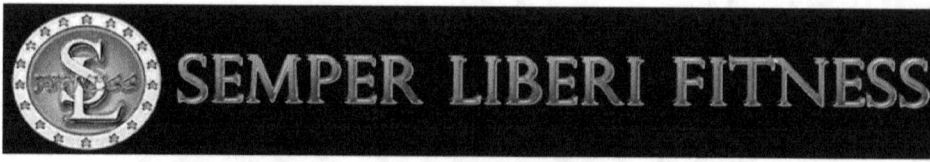

Phase: Met Con - Program 3

A1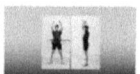

Squat with Shoulder Press
Sets: 10   Reps: 10
Tempo: Fast Rest: AsNec.

A2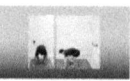

Burpee from Floor
Sets: 10   Reps: 5
Tempo: Fast Rest: AsNec

Phase: Met Con - Program 3

A1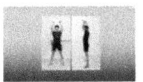

Squat with Shoulder Press
Sets: 10   Reps: 10
Tempo: Fast Rest: AsNec.

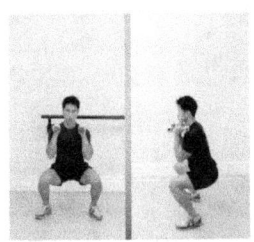 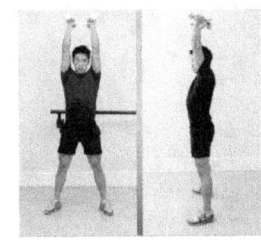

- Stand with your feet a comfortable distance apart. Take a dumbbell in each hand and hold them at shoulder height.

- Keeping your chest up, bend at your knees then hips to lower your bum down towards the ground behind you.

- Go as low as you can with control, ideally your hips should go below your knees.

- Keeping your heels on the ground, push up into the start position. Use the upward momentum to help you press the dumbbells up overhead directly above your shoulders.

- Bring the dumbbells back to the shoulder height position ready to go again.

A2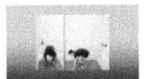

Burpee from Floor
Sets: 10   Reps: 5
Tempo: Fast Rest: AsNec

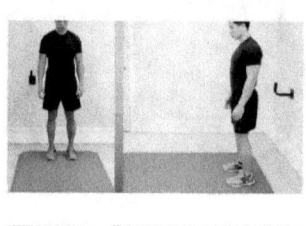 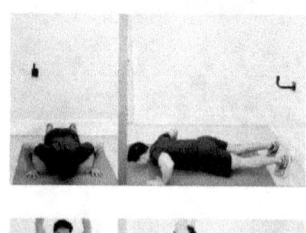

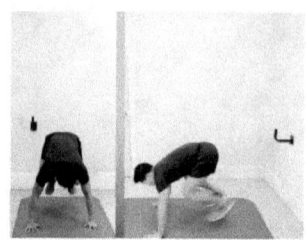 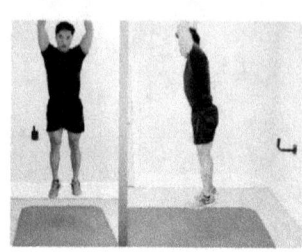

- Start standing up into a fully extended position with chest up and shoulders back and down.

- Quickly move your hands down to the floor and jump your legs back to a fully extended position while lowering your body in to the lowest position of a press up.

- Bounce your legs forward while pushing up with your arms then jump up fast and high.

- Keep your head in a neutral position throughout the movement and don't allow your hips to drop bellow the point where your body is straight from ankles to head.

Phase: Met Con - Program 4

A1 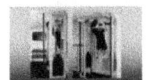 **Pull Up - Shoulder Width Grip**
Reps: 100   Tempo: Fast
Rest: AsNec

A2 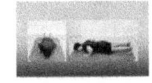 **Press Up Flat**
Reps: 100   Tempo: Fast
Rest: AsNec

A3 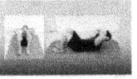 **Crunch**
Reps: 100   Tempo: Fast
Rest: AsNec

A4 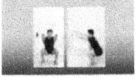 **Body Weight Squat**
Reps: 100   Tempo: Fast
Rest: AsNec

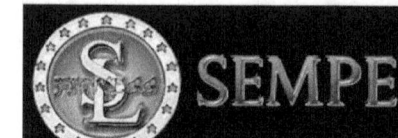
Phase: Met Con - Program 4

A1 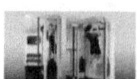 **Pull Up - Shoulder Width Grip**
Reps: 100   Tempo: Fast
Rest: AsNec

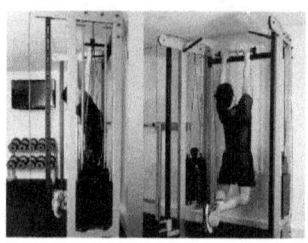 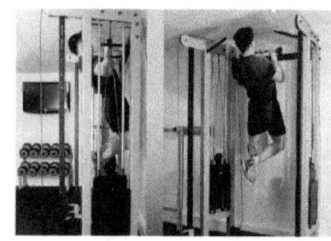

- Stand under the chin up bar at a height where you are able to grip the bar without jumping.

-Take hold of the bar with both hands facing away from you and shoulder width apart. Bring your shoulder blades back towards each other and down towards your bum.

- Pull yourself up to the top position. Your chin should be above your hands and chest pushed out.

- From the top position, lower your self down under control to the bottom.

A2 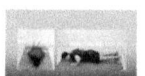 **Press Up Flat**
Reps: 100   Tempo: Fast
Rest: AsNec

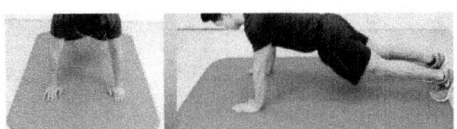 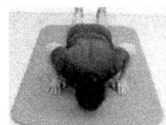 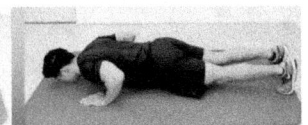

- Come down so that your hands and feet are on the floor.

- Place your hands a little wider than shoulder width apart.

- Position your hips to form a straight line from your heels to your head.

- Gently draw in your tummy using roughly 30% effort.

- Bend your elbows lowering your body toward the ground. Keep your elbows at about 45 degrees from the sides of your body.

- You should come down so that your chest is between your hands.

- Lower until your chest is a small fist away from the ground and then push back up to the start position.

A3 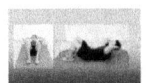 **Crunch**
Reps: 100   Tempo: Fast
Rest: AsNec

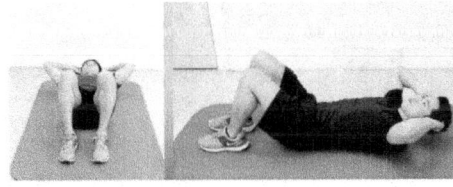 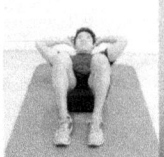 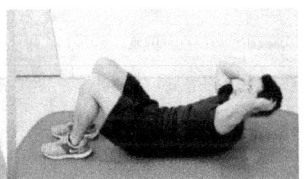

- Lie face up on a mat with knees bent and feet flat on the mat.

- Engage your core by drawing your tummy in and pelvic floor muscle (the muscle you would use to stop yourself from peeing) up with 30% effort.

- Put your tongue on the roof of your mouth, this will stop the muscles in the front of your neck overworking.

- Tuck your chin gently towards your chest and lift your shoulders and shoulder blades off the mat. Keeping your feet on the ground and core engaged; lift your torso as far towards your knees as you can.

156

- Lower back down under control so that your shoulder blades are once again on the mat.

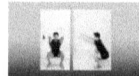

A4
Body Weight Squat
Reps: 100   Tempo: Fast
Rest: AsNec

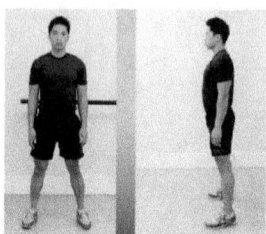 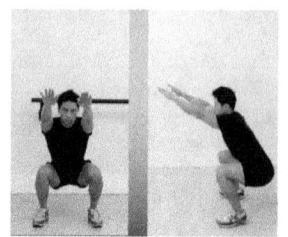

- Stand with your feet parallel and a comfortable distance apart with your weight evenly distributed between both legs.

- Keeping your chest up, bend at your knees then hips to lower your bum down towards the ground behind you.

- Go as low as you can with control, ideally your hips should go below your knees.

- Keeping your weight evenly distributed, push up as fast as you can.

Strength Program

I also want to include a portion of the strength and conditioning programs we offer to show you how they are structured and give you an idea of the type of principles we use. This is a sample beginner strength program that will help you begin a path to getting bigger and stronger.

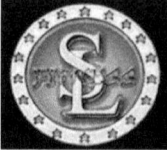
Phase: Strength-Part 1 - Program 1

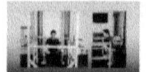

A1

Barbell Back Squat
Sets: 2   Reps: 5
Tempo: 3:1:1 Rest: 3:00
Intensity: Bar

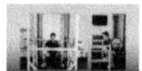

A2

Barbell Back Squat
Sets: 1   Reps: 5
Tempo: 3:1:1 Rest: 3:00
Intensity: 50%

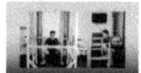

A3

Barbell Back Squat
Sets: 1   Reps: 3
Tempo: 3:1:1 Rest: 3:00
Intensity: 70%

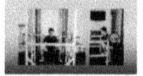

A4

Barbell Back Squat
Sets: 1   Reps: 2
Tempo: 3:1:1 Rest: 3:00
Intensity: 90%

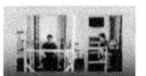

A5

Barbell Back Squat
Sets: 3   Reps: 5
Tempo: 3:1:1 Rest: 3:00
Intensity: 5RM

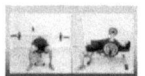

B1

Flat Bench Press - Shoulder Width Grip
Sets: 2   Reps: 5
Tempo: 1:1:3 Rest: 3:00
Intensity: Bar

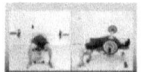

B2

Flat Bench Press - Shoulder Width Grip
Sets: 2   Reps: 5
Tempo: 1:1:3 Rest: 3:00
Intensity: 50%

B3 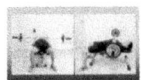 **Flat Bench Press - Shoulder Width Grip**
Sets: 2   Reps: 3
Tempo: 1:1:3 Rest: 3:00
Intensity: 70%

B4 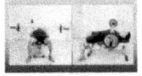 **Flat Bench Press - Shoulder Width Grip**
Sets: 2   Reps: 2
Tempo: 1:1:3 Rest: 3:00
Intensity: 90%

B5 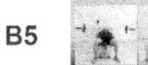 **Flat Bench Press - Shoulder Width Grip**
Sets: 2   Reps: 5
Tempo: 1:1:3 Rest: 3:00
Intensity: 5RM

C1 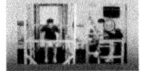 **Standing Good Morning**
Sets: 3   Reps: 10
Tempo: 3:1:1   Rest: 1:00
Intensity: 12RM

D1 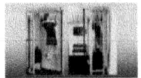 **Chin Up - Supinated Shoulder width Grip**
Sets: 3   Reps: 10
Tempo: 3:1:1   Rest: 1:00
Intensity: 12RM

Phase: Strength-Part 1 - Program 1

A1 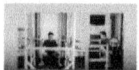 **Barbell Back Squat**
Sets: 2   Reps: 5
Tempo: 3:1:1 Rest: 3:00
Intensity: Bar

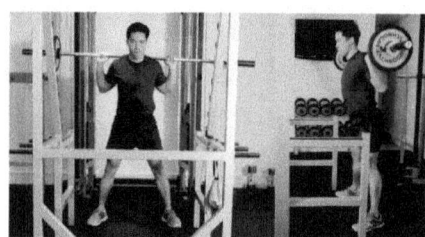 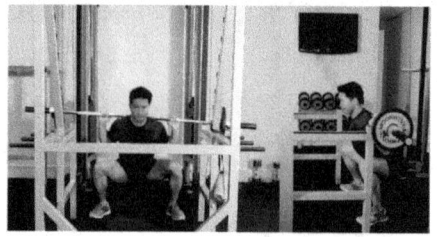

- Stand with your feet parallel and a comfortable distance apart with your weight evenly distributed between both legs.

- Take a barbell on your back, resting it evenly across your shoulders on the cushioned part of your upper back.

- Hold the bar with both hands keeping your elbows directly below your wrists.

- Keeping your chest up, bend at your knees then hips to lower your bum down towards the ground behind you.

- Go as low as you can with control, ideally your hips should go below your knees. Keeping your heels on the ground, push up into the start position.

A2 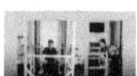 **Barbell Back Squat**
Sets: 1   Reps: 5

Tempo: 3:1:1 Rest: 3:00
Intensity: 50%

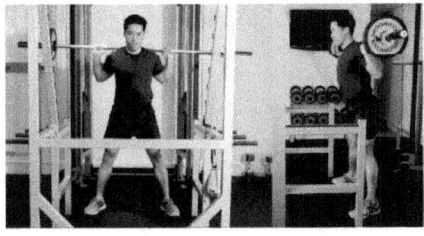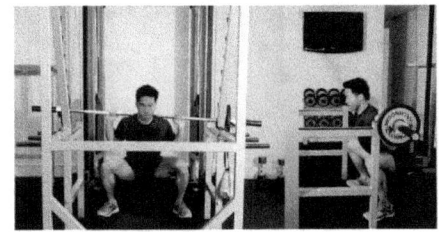

- Stand with your feet parallel and a comfortable distance apart with your weight evenly distributed between both legs.

- Take a barbell on your back, resting it evenly across your shoulders on the cushioned part of your upper back.

- Hold the bar with both hands keeping your elbows directly below your wrists.

- Keeping your chest up, bend at your knees then hips to lower your bum down towards the ground behind you.

- Go as low as you can with control, ideally your hips should go below your knees. Keeping your heels on the ground, push up into the start position.

A3 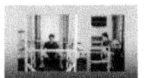 **Barbell Back Squat**
Sets: 1   Reps: 3
Tempo: 3:1:1 Rest: 3:00
Intensity: 70%

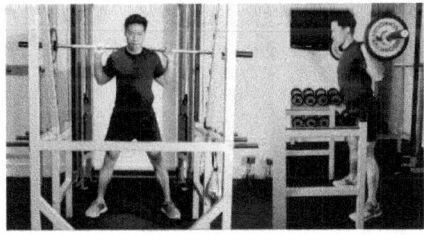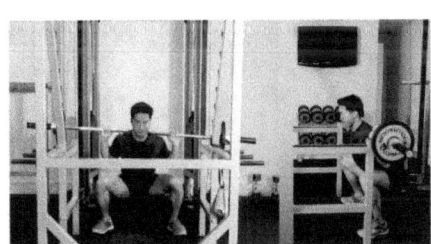

- Stand with your feet parallel and a comfortable distance apart with your weight evenly distributed between both legs.

- Take a barbell on your back, resting it evenly across your shoulders on the cushioned part of your upper back.

- Hold the bar with both hands keeping your elbows directly below your wrists.

- Keeping your chest up, bend at your knees then hips to lower your bum down towards the ground behind you.

- Go as low as you can with control, ideally your hips should go below your knees. Keeping your heels on the ground, push up into the start position.

A4 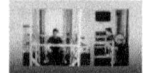 **Barbell Back Squat**
Sets: 1   Reps: 2
Tempo: 3:1:1   Rest: 3:00
Intensity: 90%

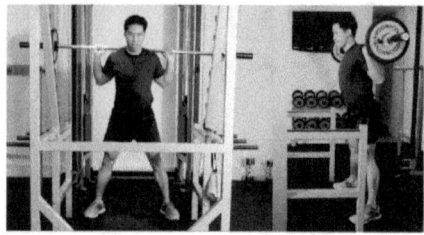 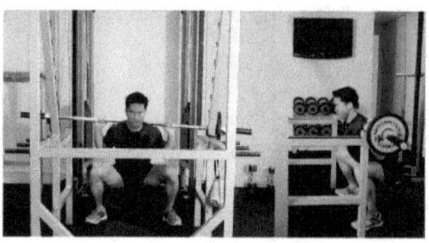

- Stand with your feet parallel and a comfortable distance apart with your weight evenly distributed between both legs.

- Take a barbell on your back, resting it evenly across your shoulders on the cushioned part of your upper back.

- Hold the bar with both hands keeping your elbows directly below your wrists.

- Keeping your chest up, bend at your knees then hips to lower your bum down towards the ground behind you.

- Go as low as you can with control, ideally your hips should go below your knees. Keeping your heels on the ground, push up into the start position.

A5 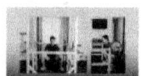 **Barbell Back Squat**
Sets: 3   Reps: 5
Tempo: 3:1:1   Rest: 3:00
Intensity: 5RM

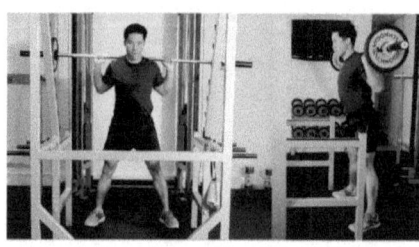 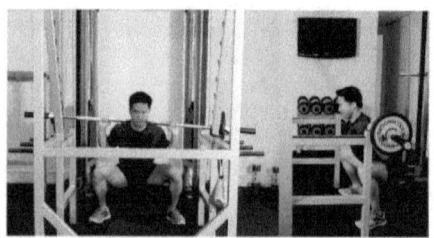

163

- Stand with your feet parallel and a comfortable distance apart with your weight evenly distributed between both legs.

- Take a barbell on your back, resting it evenly across your shoulders on the cushioned part of your upper back.

- Hold the bar with both hands keeping your elbows directly below your wrists.

- Keeping your chest up, bend at your knees then hips to lower your bum down towards the ground behind you.

- Go as low as you can with control, ideally your hips should go below your knees. Keeping your heels on the ground, push up into the start position.

B1 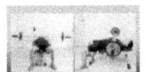 **Flat Bench Press - Shoulder Width Grip**
Sets: 2   Reps: 5
Tempo: 1:1:3 Rest: 3:00
Intensity: Bar

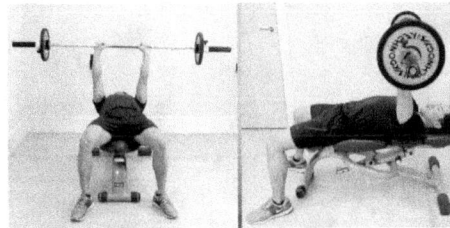 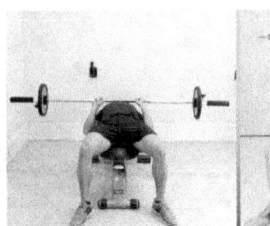 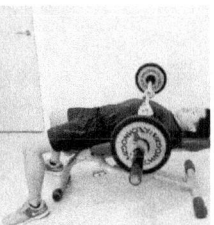

- Lie face up on a bench. Place your hands shoulder width apart on the bar.

- Take the weight and bring it slightly forward so it sits over your chest.

- Lower the bar under control down towards your chest.

- As the bar touches your chest lift back up to the top position.

- keep your bum, back and head in contact with the bench at all times.

B2 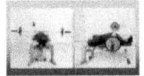 **Flat Bench Press - Shoulder Width Grip**
Sets: 2   Reps: 5
Tempo: 1:1:3 Rest: 3:00
Intensity: 50%

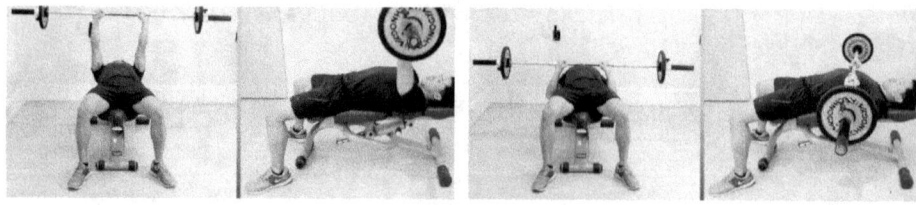

- Lie face up on a bench. Place your hands shoulder width apart on the bar.

- Take the weight and bring it slightly forward so it sits over your chest.

- Lower the bar under control down towards your chest.

- As the bar touches your chest lift back up to the top position.

- keep your bum, back and head in contact with the bench at all times.

B3 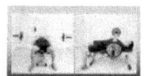   **Flat Bench Press - Shoulder Width Grip**
Sets: 2   Reps: 3
Tempo: 1:1:3 Rest: 3:00
Intensity: 70%

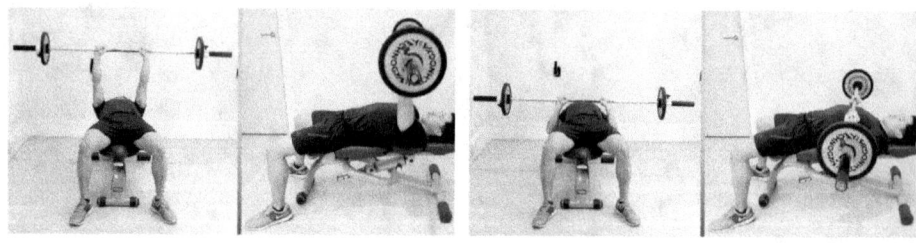

- Lie face up on a bench. Place your hands shoulder width apart on the bar.

- Take the weight and bring it slightly forward so it sits over your chest.

- Lower the bar under control down towards your chest.

- As the bar touches your chest lift back up to the top position.

- keep your bum, back and head in contact with the bench at all times.

B4 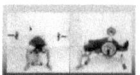   **Flat Bench Press - Shoulder Width Grip**
Sets: 2   Reps: 2

Intensity 90%

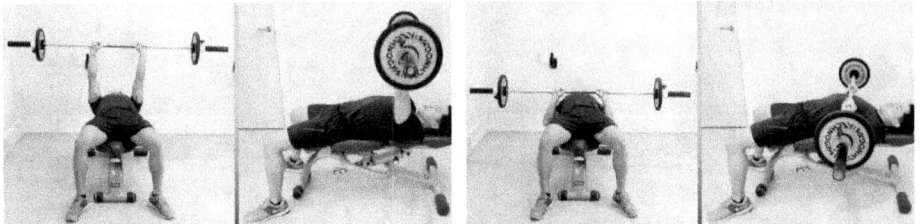

- Lie face up on a bench. Place your hands shoulder width apart on the bar.

- Take the weight and bring it slightly forward so it sits over your chest.

- Lower the bar under control down towards your chest.

- As the bar touches your chest lift back up to the top position.

- keep your bum, back and head in contact with the bench at all times.

B5 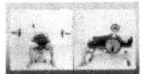 **Flat Bench Press - Shoulder Width Grip**
Sets: 2   Reps: 5
Tempo: 1:1:3   Rest: 3:00
Intensity: 5RM

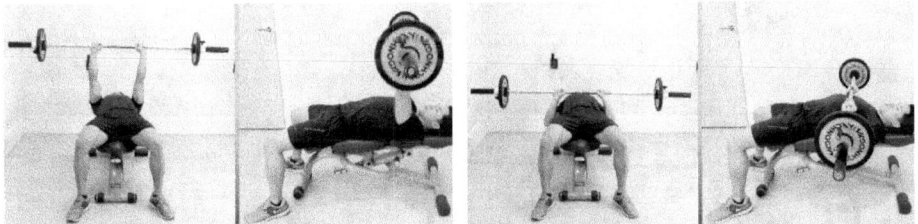

- Lie face up on a bench. Place your hands shoulder width apart on the bar.

- Take the weight and bring it slightly forward so it sits over your chest.

- Lower the bar under control down towards your chest.

- As the bar touches your chest lift back up to the top position.

- keep your bum, back and head in contact with the bench at all times.

C1 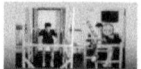 **Standing Good Morning**
Sets: 3   Reps: 10
Tempo: 3:1:1   Rest: 1:00
Intensity: 12RM

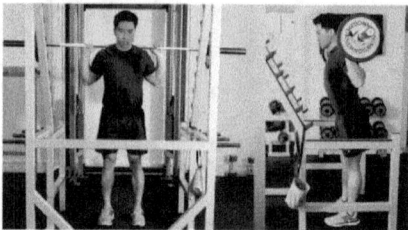 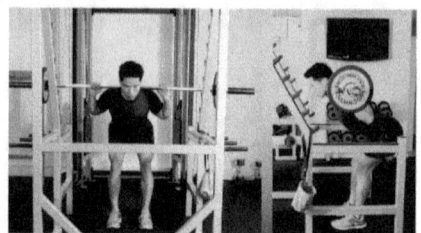

- Take a Barbell on your back, resting it evenly across your shoulders and the cushioned part of your upper back.

- Stand up straight, push your chest out and hollow your lower back.

- Lean forward from your hips as far as you comfortably can. Keep your chest out and back hollowed.

- Lift back up until your upper body is once again in an upright position.

D1 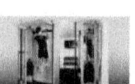 **Chin Up - Supinated Shoulder width Grip**
Sets: 3   Reps: 10
Tempo: 3:1:1   Rest: 1:00
Intensity: 12RM

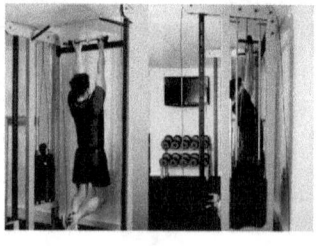 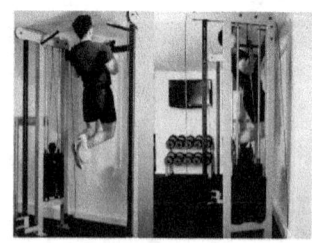

- Stand under the chin up bar at a height where you are able to grip the bar without jumping.

-Take hold of the bar with both hands facing you and shoulder width apart. Bring your shoulder blades back towards each other and down towards your bum.

- Pull yourself up to the top position. Your chin should be above your hands and chest pushed out.

- From the top position, lower your self down under control to the bottom

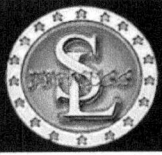

SEMPER LIBERI FITNESS

Phase: Strength-Part 1 - Program 2

A1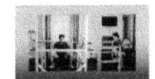
Barbell Back Squat
Sets: 2   Reps: 5
Tempo: 3:1:1 Rest: 3:00
Intensity: Bar

A2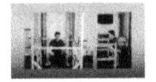
Barbell Back Squat
Sets: 1   Reps: 5
Tempo: 3:1:1 Rest: 3:00
Intensity: 50%

A3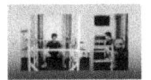
Barbell Back Squat
Sets: 1   Reps: 3
Tempo: 3:1:1 Rest: 3:00
Intensity: 70%

A4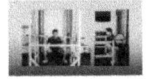
Barbell Back Squat
Sets: 1   Reps: 2
Tempo: 3:1:1 Rest: 3:00
Intensity: 90%

A5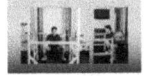
Barbell Back Squat
Sets: 3   Reps: 5
Tempo: 3:1:1 Rest: 3:00
Intensity: 5RM

B1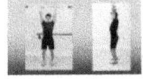
Standing Shoulder Press - Barbell - Shoulder Width Grip
Sets: 2   Reps: 5
Tempo: 1:1:3 Rest: 3:00
Intensity: Bar

B2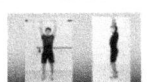
Standing Shoulder Press - Barbell - Shoulder Width Grip
Sets: 1   Reps: 5
Tempo: 1:1:3 Rest: 3:00

Intensity: 50%

B3 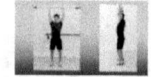 **Standing Shoulder Press - Barbell - Shoulder Width Grip**
Sets: 1   Reps: 3
Tempo: 1:1:3   Rest: 3:00
Intensity: 70%

B4 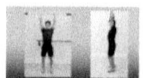 **Standing Shoulder Press - Barbell - Shoulder Width Grip**
Sets: 1   Reps: 2
Tempo: 1:1:3   Rest: 3:00
Intensity: 90%

B5 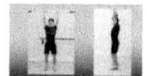 **Standing Shoulder Press - Barbell - Shoulder Width Grip**
Sets: 3   Reps: 5
Tempo: 1:1:3   Rest: 3:00
Intensity: 5RM

C1 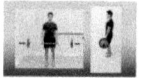 **Dead Lift from Floor Clean Grip**
Sets: 2   Reps: 5
Tempo: 1:1:3 Rest: 3:00
Intensity: Bar

C2 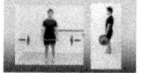 **Dead Lift from Floor Clean Grip**
Sets: 1   Reps: 5
Tempo: 1:1:3   Rest: 3:00
Intensity: 50%

C3 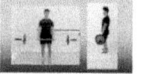 **Dead Lift from Floor Clean Grip**
Sets: 1   Reps: 3
Tempo: 1:1:3   Rest: 3:00
Intensity: 70%

C4 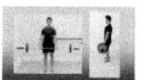 **Dead Lift from Floor Clean Grip**
Sets: 1   Reps: 2
Tempo: 1:1:3   Rest: 3:00
Intensity: 90%

C5 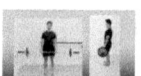 **Dead Lift from Floor Clean Grip**
Sets: 1   Reps: 5
Tempo: 1:1:3   Rest: 3:00
Intensity: 5RM

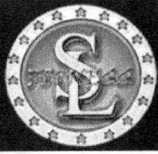

SEMPER LIBERI FITNESS

Phase: Strength-Part 1 - Program 2

A1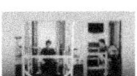
Barbell Back Squat
Sets: 2   Reps: 5
Tempo: 3:1:1 Rest: 3:00
Intensity: Bar

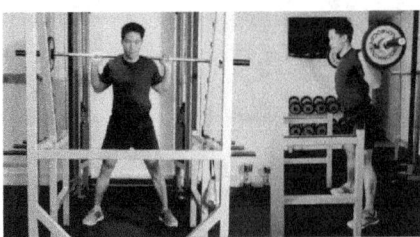 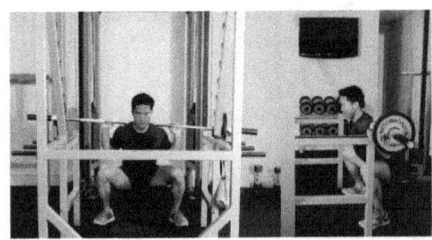

- Stand with your feet parallel and a comfortable distance apart with your weight evenly distributed between both legs.

- Take a barbell on your back, resting it evenly across your shoulders on the cushioned part of your upper back.

- Hold the bar with both hands keeping your elbows directly below your wrists.

- Keeping your chest up, bend at your knees then hips to lower your bum down towards the ground behind you.

- Go as low as you can with control, ideally your hips should go below your knees. Keeping your heels on the ground, push up into the start position.

A2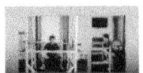
Barbell Back Squat
Sets: 1   Reps: 5

Tempo: 3:1:1 Rest: 3:00
Intensity: 50%

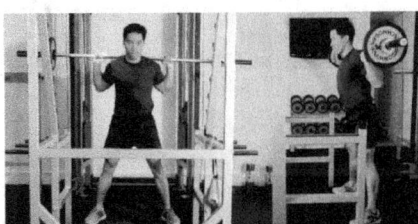 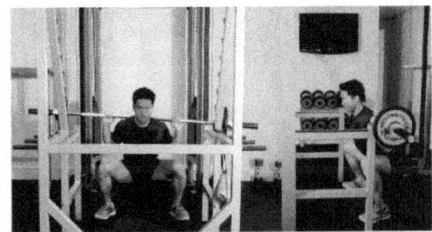

- Go as low as you can with control, ideally your hips should go below your knees. Keeping your heels on the ground, push up into the start position.

A4 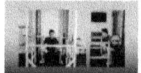 **Barbell Back Squat**
Sets: 1   Reps: 2
Tempo: 3:1:1 Rest: 3:00
Intensity: 90%

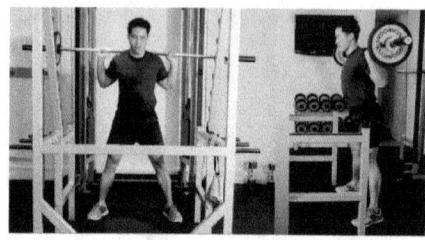 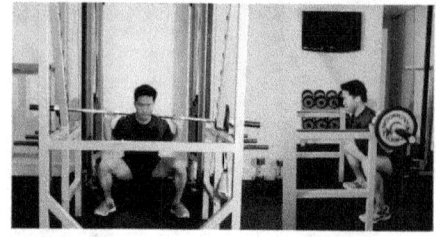

- Stand with your feet parallel and a comfortable distance apart with your weight evenly distributed between both legs.

- Take a barbell on your back, resting it evenly across your shoulders on the cushioned part of your upper back.

- Hold the bar with both hands keeping your elbows directly below your wrists.

- Keeping your chest up, bend at your knees then hips to lower your bum down towards the ground behind you.

- Go as low as you can with control, ideally your hips should go below your knees. Keeping your heels on the ground, push up into the start position.

A5 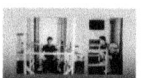 **Barbell Back Squat**
Sets: 3   Reps: 5
Tempo: 3:1:1 Rest: 3:00
Intensity: 5RM

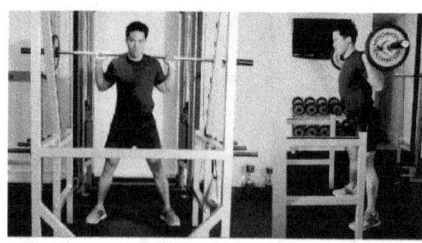 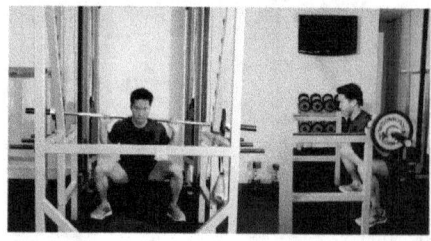

- Stand with your feet parallel and a comfortable distance apart with your weight evenly distributed between both legs.

- Take a barbell on your back, resting it evenly across your shoulders on the cushioned part of your upper back.

- Hold the bar with both hands keeping your elbows directly below your wrists.

- Keeping your chest up, bend at your knees then hips to lower your bum down towards the ground behind you.

- Go as low as you can with control, ideally your hips should go below your knees. Keeping your heels on the ground, push up into the start position.

B1 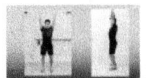 **Standing Shoulder Press - Barbell - Shoulder Width Grip**
Sets: 2   Reps: 5
Tempo: 1:1:3 Rest: 3:00
Intensity: Bar

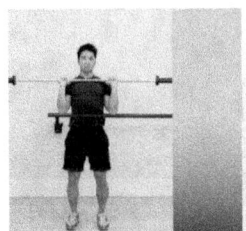 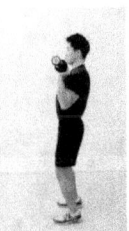 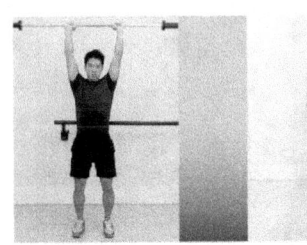 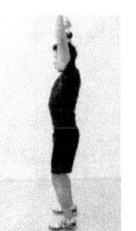

- Stand with your feet hip width apart, tummy gently drawn in with about 30% effort and your shoulders back and down. Take the barbell with a shoulder width grip at shoulder height with your palms facing away from you.

- Keeping your core engaged and body upright push up above your shoulders to a straight arm position.

- Lower under control to the start position.

B2 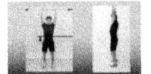 **Standing Shoulder Press - Barbell - Shoulder Width Grip**
Sets: 1   Reps: 5
Tempo: 1:1:3 Rest: 3:00
Intensity: 50%

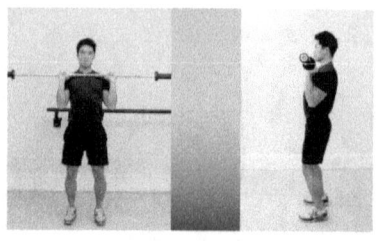 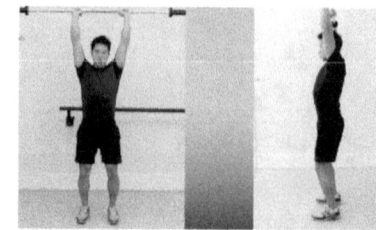

- Stand with your feet hip width apart, tummy gently drawn in with about 30% effort and your shoulders back and down. Take the barbell with a shoulder width grip at shoulder height with your palms facing away from you.

- Keeping your core engaged and body upright push up above your shoulders to a straight arm position.

- Lower under control to the start position.

B3 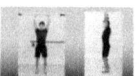 **Standing Shoulder Press - Barbell - Shoulder Width Grip**
Sets: 1   Reps: 3
Tempo: 1:1:3 Rest: 3:00
Intensity: 70%

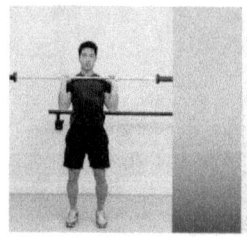 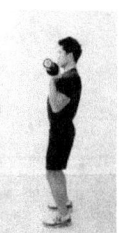 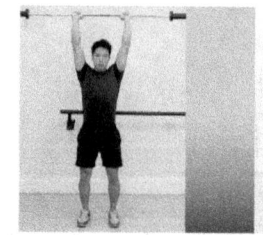 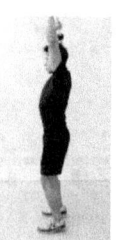

- Stand with your feet hip width apart, tummy gently drawn in with about 30% effort and your shoulders back and down. Take the barbell with a shoulder width grip at shoulder height with your palms facing away from you.

- Keeping your core engaged and body upright push up above your shoulders to a straight arm position.

- Lower under control to the start position.

B4 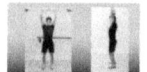 **Standing Shoulder Press - Barbell - Shoulder Width Grip**
Sets: 1   Reps: 2
Tempo: 1:1:3 Rest: 3:00
Intensity: 90%

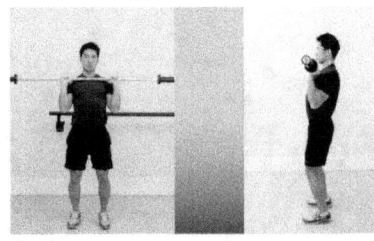 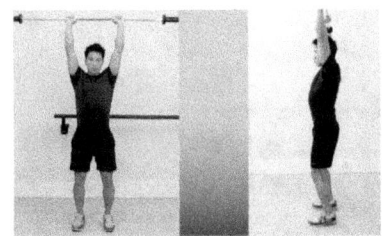

- Stand with your feet hip width apart, tummy gently drawn in with about 30% effort and your shoulders back and down. Take the barbell with a shoulder width grip at shoulder height with your palms facing away from you.

- Keeping your core engaged and body upright push up above your shoulders to a straight arm position.

- Lower under control to the start position.

B5 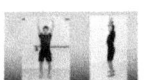 **Standing Shoulder Press - Barbell - Shoulder Width Grip**
Sets: 3   Reps: 5
Tempo: 1:1:3   Rest: 3:00
Intensity: 5RM

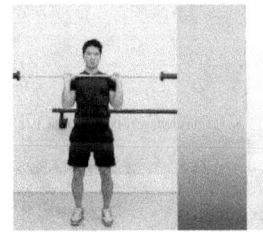 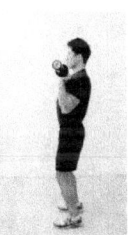 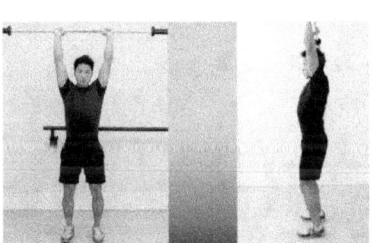

- Stand with your feet hip width apart, tummy gently drawn in with about 30% effort and your shoulders back and down. Take the barbell with a shoulder width grip at shoulder height with your palms facing away from you.

- Keeping your core engaged and body upright push up above your shoulders to a straight arm position.

- Lower under control to the start position.

C1 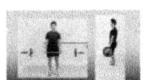 **Dead Lift from Floor Clean Grip**
Sets: 2   Reps: 5
Tempo: 1:1:3 Rest: 3:00
Intensity: Bar

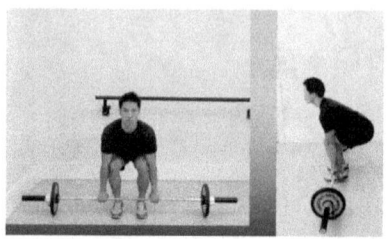 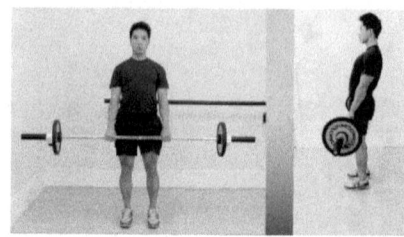

- Start standing with your toes under the bar.

- Lean over, bend your knees and take hold of the bar with your hands a little wider than your knees and palms facing you.

- Push your chest out and hollow your lower back. Gently draw in your tummy with approximately 30% effort.

- Pushing through your feet and keeping your low back hollowed with your chest pushed out, lift the bar until you are standing in an upright position.

- Keeping your low back hollowed with your chest pushed out; lower the bar in a controlled manner down to the floor.

C2 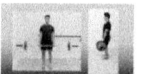 **Dead Lift from Floor Clean Grip**
Sets: 1   Reps: 5
Tempo: 1:1:3 Rest: 3:00
Intensity: 50%

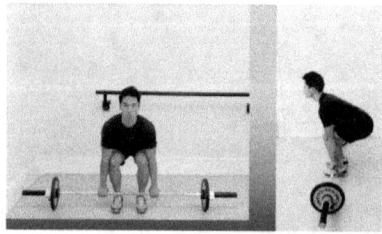 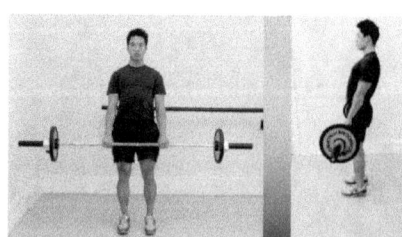

- Start standing with your toes under the bar.

- Lean over, bend your knees and take hold of the bar with your hands a little wider than your knees and palms facing you.

- Push your chest out and hollow your lower back. Gently draw in your tummy with approximately 30% effort.

- Pushing through your feet and keeping your low back hollowed with your chest pushed out, lift the bar until you are standing in an upright position.

- Keeping your low back hollowed with your chest pushed out; lower the bar in a controlled manner down to the floor.

C3 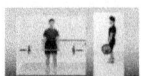 **Dead Lift from Floor Clean Grip**
Sets: 1   Reps: 3
Tempo: 1:1:3 Rest: 3:00
Intensity: 70%

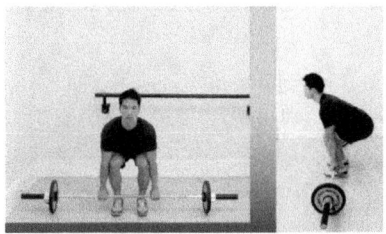 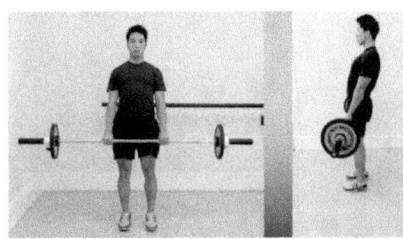

- Start standing with your toes under the bar.

- Lean over, bend your knees and take hold of the bar with your hands a little wider than your knees and palms facing you.

- Push your chest out and hollow your lower back. Gently draw in your tummy with approximately 30% effort.

- Pushing through your feet and keeping your low back hollowed with your chest pushed out, lift the bar until you are standing in an upright position.

- Keeping your low back hollowed with your chest pushed out; lower the bar in a controlled manner down to the floor.

C4 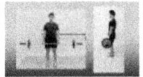 **Dead Lift from Floor Clean Grip**
Sets: 1   Reps: 2
Tempo: 1:1:3 Rest: 3:00
Intensity: 90%

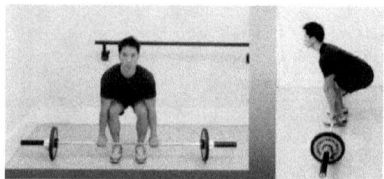 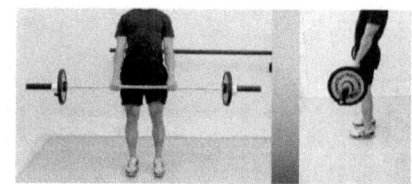

- Start standing with your toes under the bar.

- Lean over, bend your knees and take hold of the bar with your hands a little wider than your knees and palms facing you.

- Push your chest out and hollow your lower back. Gently draw in your tummy with approximately 30% effort.

- Pushing through your feet and keeping your low back hollowed with your chest pushed out, lift the bar until you are standing in an upright position.

- Keeping your low back hollowed with your chest pushed out; lower the bar in a controlled manner down to the floor.

C5 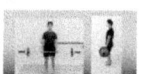 **Dead Lift from Floor Clean Grip**
Sets: 1   Reps: 5
Tempo: 1:1:3   Rest: 3:00
Intensity: 5RM

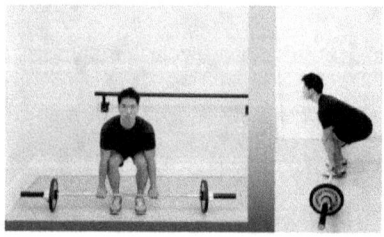 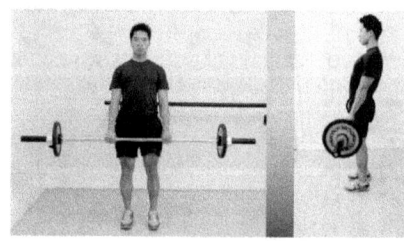

- Start standing with your toes under the bar.

- Lean over, bend your knees and take hold of the bar with your hands a little wider than your knees and palms facing you.

- Push your chest out and hollow your lower back. Gently draw in your tummy with approximately 30% effort.

- Pushing through your feet and keeping your low back hollowed with your chest pushed out, lift the bar until you are standing in an upright position.

- Keeping your low back hollowed with your chest pushed out; lower the bar in a controlled manner down to the floor.

Phase: Strength-Part 1 - Program 3

A1
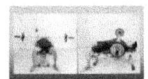
Flat Bench Press - Shoulder Width Grip
Sets: 2   Reps: 5
Tempo: 1:1:3 Rest: 3:00
Intensity: Bar

A2
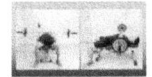
Flat Bench Press - Shoulder Width Grip
Sets: 1   Reps: 5
Tempo: 1:1:3 Rest: 3:00
Intensity: 50%

A3
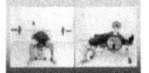
Flat Bench Press - Shoulder Width Grip
Sets: 1   Reps: 3
Tempo: 1:1:3 Rest: 3:00
Intensity: 70%

A4
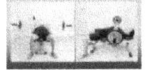
Flat Bench Press - Shoulder Width Grip
Sets: 1   Reps: 2
Tempo: 1:1:3 Rest: 3:00
Intensity: 90%

A5
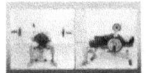
Flat Bench Press - Shoulder Width Grip
Sets: 3   Reps: 5
Tempo: 1:1:3 Rest: 3:00
Intensity: 5RM

B1
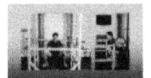
Barbell Back Squat
Sets: 2   Reps: 5
Tempo: 3:1:1 Rest: 3:00
Intensity: Bar

B2
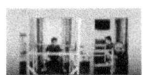
Barbell Back Squat
Sets: 1   Reps: 5
Tempo: 3:1:1 Rest: 3:00
Intensity: 50%

B3 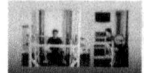 **Barbell Back Squat**
Sets: 1   Reps: 3
Tempo: 3:1:1 Rest: 3:00
Intensity: 70%

B4 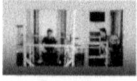 **Barbell Back Squat**
Sets: 1   Reps: 2
Tempo: 3:1:1 Rest: 3:00
Intensity: 90%

B5 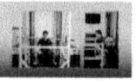 **Barbell Back Squat**
Sets: 3   Reps: 5
Tempo: 3:1:1 Rest: 3:00
Intensity: 5RM

C1 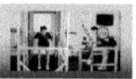 **Standing Good Morning**
Sets: 3   Reps: 10
Tempo: 3:1:1   Rest: 1:00
Intensity: 12RM

D1 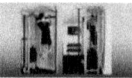 **Chin Up - Supinated Shoulder width Grip**
Sets: 3   Reps: 10
Tempo: 3:1:1   Rest: 1:00
Intensity: 12RM

Phase: Strength-Part 1 - Program 3

A1 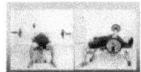 **Flat Bench Press - Shoulder Width Grip**
Sets: 2 Reps: 5
Tempo: 1:1:3 Rest: 3:00
Intensity: Bar

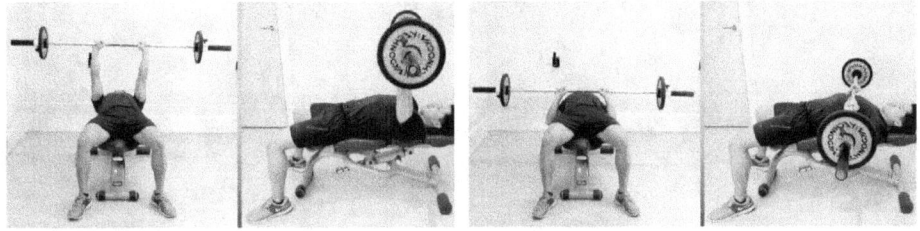

- Lie face up on a bench. Place your hands shoulder width apart on the bar.

- Take the weight and bring it slightly forward so it sits over your chest.

- Lower the bar under control down towards your chest.

- As the bar touches your chest lift back up to the top position.

- keep your bum, back and head in contact with the bench at all times.

A2 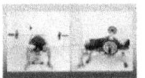 **Flat Bench Press - Shoulder Width Grip**
Sets: 1 Reps: 5
Tempo: 1:1:3 Rest: 3:00
Intensity: 50%

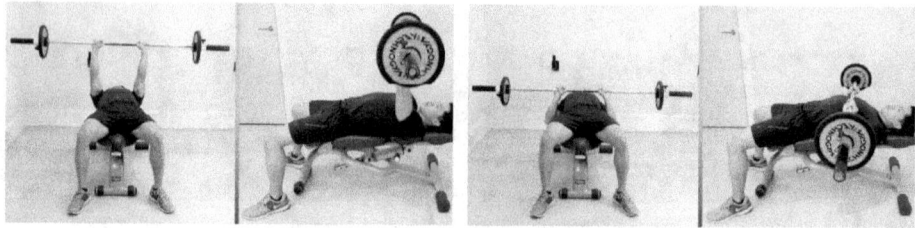

- Lie face up on a bench. Place your hands shoulder width apart on the bar.

- Take the weight and bring it slightly forward so it sits over your chest.

- Lower the bar under control down towards your chest.

- As the bar touches your chest lift back up to the top position.

- keep your bum, back and head in contact with the bench at all times.

A3 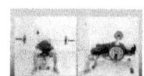 **Flat Bench Press - Shoulder Width Grip**
Sets: 1   Reps: 3
Tempo: 1:1:3 Rest: 3:00
Intensity: 70%

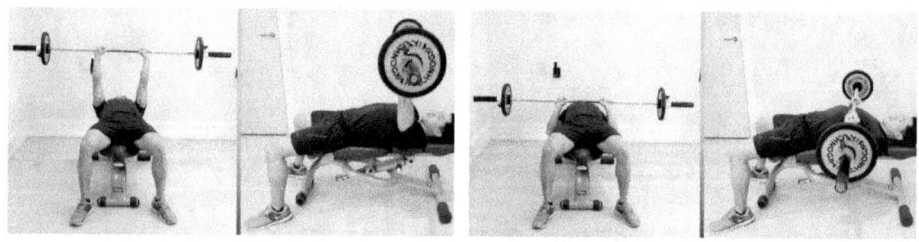

- Lie face up on a bench. Place your hands shoulder width apart on the bar.

- Take the weight and bring it slightly forward so it sits over your chest.

- Lower the bar under control down towards your chest.

- As the bar touches your chest lift back up to the top position.

- keep your bum, back and head in contact with the bench at all times.

A4 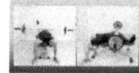 **Flat Bench Press - Shoulder Width Grip**
Sets: 1   Reps: 2
Tempo: 1:1:3 Rest: 3:00
Intensity: 90%

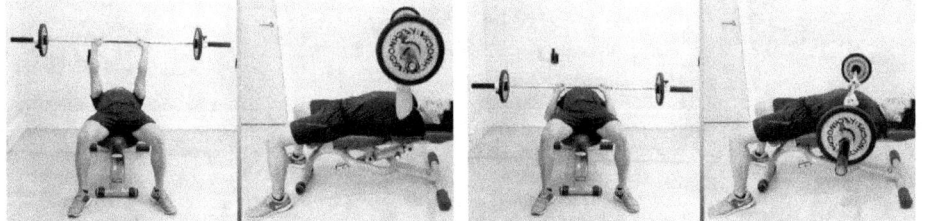

- Lie face up on a bench. Place your hands shoulder width apart on the bar.

- Take the weight and bring it slightly forward so it sits over your chest.

- Lower the bar under control down towards your chest.

- As the bar touches your chest lift back up to the top position.

- keep your bum, back and head in contact with the bench at all times.

A5 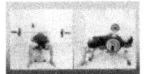 **Flat Bench Press - Shoulder Width Grip**
Sets: 3   Reps: 5
Tempo: 1:1:3   Rest: 3:00
Intensity: 5RM

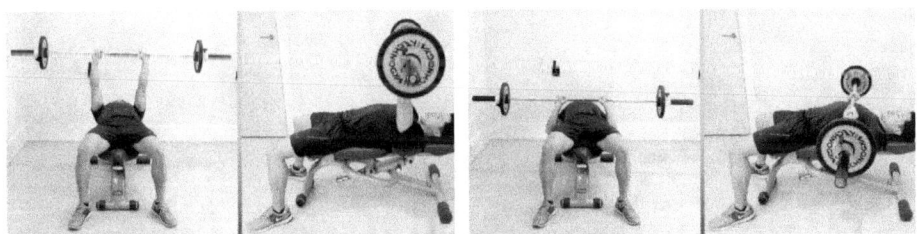

- Lie face up on a bench. Place your hands shoulder width apart on the bar.

- Take the weight and bring it slightly forward so it sits over your chest.

- Lower the bar under control down towards your chest.

- As the bar touches your chest lift back up to the top position.

- keep your bum, back and head in contact with the bench at all times.

B1 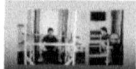 **Barbell Back Squat**
Sets: 2   Reps: 5
Tempo: 3:1:1 Rest: 3:00
Intensity: Bar

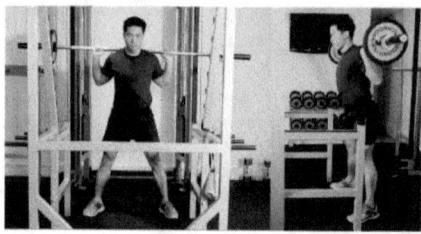 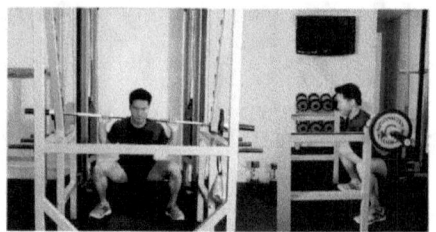

- Stand with your feet parallel and a comfortable distance apart with your weight evenly distributed between both legs.

- Take a barbell on your back, resting it evenly across your shoulders on the cushioned part of your upper back.

- Hold the bar with both hands keeping your elbows directly below your wrists.

- Keeping your chest up, bend at your knees then hips to lower your bum down towards the ground behind you.

- Go as low as you can with control, ideally your hips should go below your knees. Keeping your heels on the ground, push up into the start position.

B2 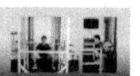 **Barbell Back Squat**
Sets: 1   Reps: 5
Tempo: 3:1:1   Rest: 3:00

Intensity: 50%

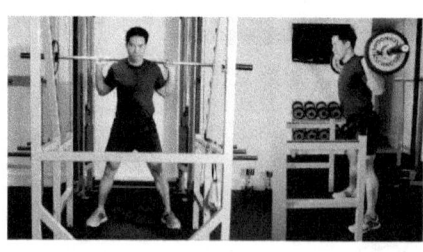 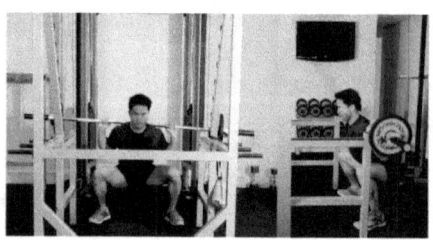

- Stand with your feet parallel and a comfortable distance apart with your weight evenly distributed between both legs.

- Take a barbell on your back, resting it evenly across your shoulders on the cushioned part of your upper back.

- Hold the bar with both hands keeping your elbows directly below your wrists.

- Keeping your chest up, bend at your knees then hips to lower your bum down towards the ground behind you.

- Go as low as you can with control, ideally your hips should go below your knees. Keeping your heels on the ground, push up into the start position.

B3 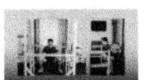 **Barbell Back Squat**
Sets: 1   Reps: 3
Tempo: 3:1:1 Rest: 3:00
Intensity: 70%

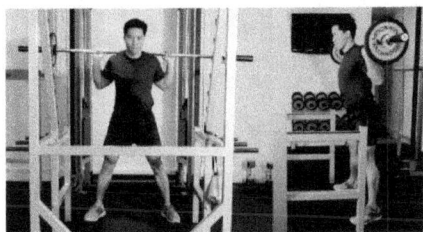 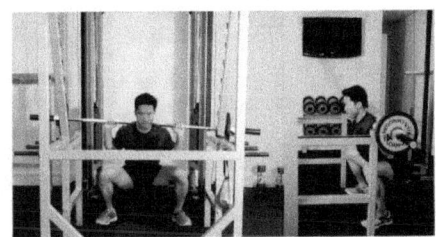

- Stand with your feet parallel and a comfortable distance apart with your weight evenly distributed between both legs.

- Take a barbell on your back, resting it evenly across your shoulders on the cushioned part of your upper back.

- Hold the bar with both hands keeping your elbows directly below your wrists.

- Keeping your chest up, bend at your knees then hips to lower your bum down towards the ground behind you.

- Go as low as you can with control, ideally your hips should go below your knees. Keeping your heels on the ground, push up into the start position.

B4 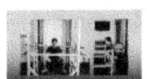 **Barbell Back Squat**
Sets: 1   Reps: 2
Tempo: 3:1:1 Rest: 3:00
Intensity: 90%

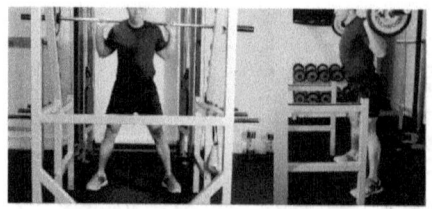 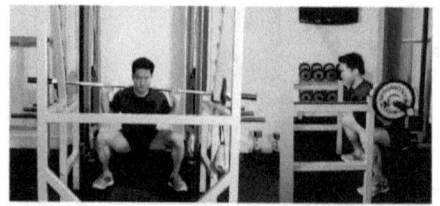

- Stand with your feet parallel and a comfortable distance apart with your weight evenly distributed between both legs.

- Take a barbell on your back, resting it evenly across your shoulders on the cushioned part of your upper back.

- Hold the bar with both hands keeping your elbows directly below your wrists.

- Keeping your chest up, bend at your knees then hips to lower your bum down towards the ground behind you.

- Go as low as you can with control, ideally your hips should go below your knees. Keeping your heels on the ground, push up into the start position.

B5 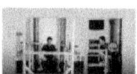 **Barbell Back Squat**
Sets: 3   Reps: 5
Tempo: 3:1:1 Rest: 3:00
Intensity: 5RM

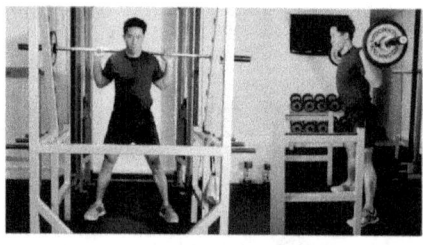 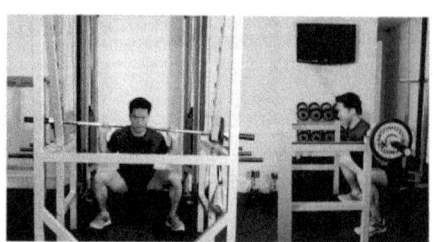

- Stand with your feet parallel and a comfortable distance apart with your weight evenly distributed between both legs.

- Take a barbell on your back, resting it evenly across your shoulders on the cushioned part of your upper back.

- Hold the bar with both hands keeping your elbows directly below your wrists.

- Keeping your chest up, bend at your knees then hips to lower your bum down towards the ground behind you.

- Go as low as you can with control, ideally your hips should go below your knees. Keeping your heels on the ground, push up into the start position.

C1 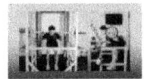 **Standing Good Morning**
Sets: 3   Reps: 10
Tempo: 3:1:1   Rest: 1:00
Intensity: 12RM

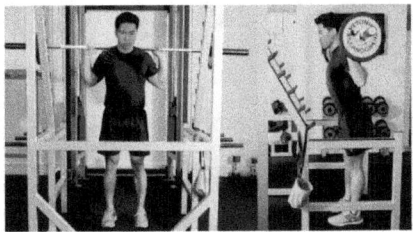 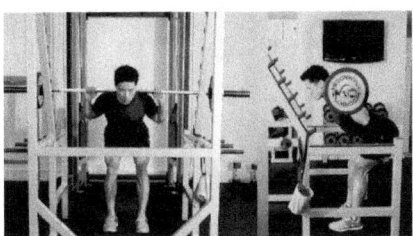

- Take a Barbell on your back, resting it evenly across your shoulders and the cushioned part of your upper back.

- Stand up straight, push your chest out and hollow your lower back.

- Lean forward from your hips as far as you comfortably can. Keep your chest out and back hollowed.

- Lift back up until your upper body is once again in an upright position.

D1 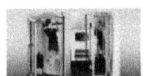 **Chin Up - Supinated Shoulder width Grip**
Sets: 3   Reps: 10
Tempo: 3:1:1   Rest: 1:00
Intensity: 12RM

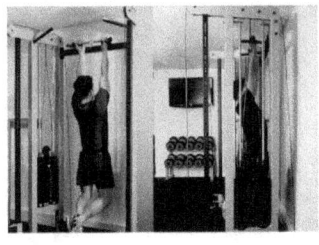 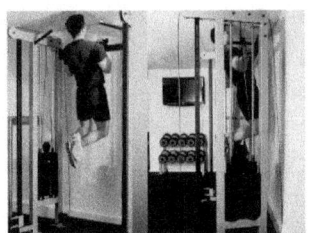

- Stand under the chin up bar at a height where you are able to grip the bar without jumping.

-Take hold of the bar with both hands facing you and shoulder width apart. Bring your shoulder blades back towards each other and down towards your bum.

- Pull yourself up to the top position. Your chin should be above your hands and chest pushed out.

- From the top position, lower your self down under control to the bottom.

Fat Loss

This is a beginner fat loss program based on our conditioning principles. This is similar to the other fat loss programs we have available on our site. We have a growing library available to ensure you continue to see success.

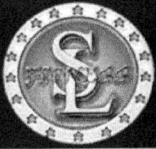

SEMPER LIBERI FITNESS

Phase: Fat Loss - Beginner - Program 1

A1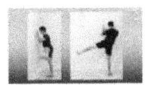
Swinging Adductor Stretch
Sets: 1   Reps: 10
Tempo: Med

A2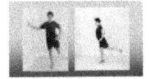
Swinging Hamstring Stretch
Sets: 1   Reps: 10
Tempo: Med

A3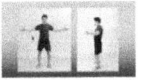
Swinging Pectoral Stretch
Sets: 1   Reps: 10
Tempo: Med

A4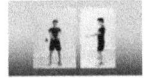
Arm Circles
Sets: 1   Reps: 10
Tempo: Med

A5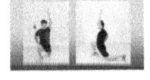
Lunging Hip Flexor Stretch
Sets: 1   Reps: 10
Tempo: Med

B1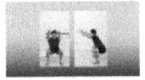
Metabolic Squat
Sets: 3   Reps: 12
Tempo: Med   Rest: 30sec
Intensity: 15RM

C1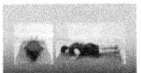
Press Up Flat
Sets: 3   Reps: 12
Tempo: Med   Rest: 30sec
Intensity: 15RM

D1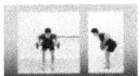
Bent over Row, Dumbbells - Pronated Grip
Sets: 3   Reps: 12
Tempo: Med   Rest: 30sec
Intensity: 15RM

E1 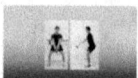 **2 Arm Single Kettlebell Swing**
Sets: 3   Reps: 12
Tempo: Med   Rest: 30sec
Intensity: 15RM

F1 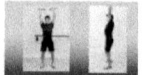 **Standing Shoulder Press - Dumbbells - Pronated Grip**
Sets: 3   Reps: 12
Tempo: Med   Rest: 30sec
Intensity: 15RM

G1 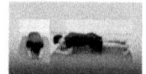 **Plank**
Sets: 3   Reps: 12
Tempo: Med   Rest: 30sec
Intensity: 15RM

H1 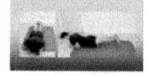 **Foam Roll Quadriceps**
Tempo: 1-2min

H2 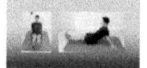 **Foam Roll Hamstrings**
Tempo: 1-2min

H3 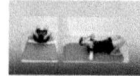 **Foam Roll Thoracic**
Tempo: 1-2min

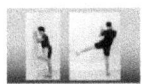

Phase: Fat Loss - Beginner - Program 1

A1 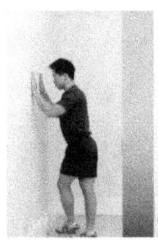 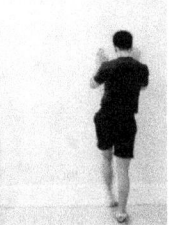 **Swinging Adductor Stretch**
Sets: 1 Reps: 10
Tempo: Med

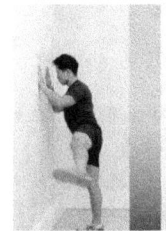 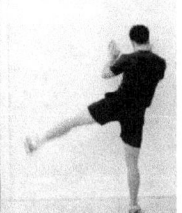

- Stand with feet hip width apart and hands on a wall for support.

- Swing one leg out to the side slightly stretching the inside of that leg.

- Swing the same leg across your body out to the other side.

- Repeat the movement gradually increasing the stretch each time.

- Complete all your reps on one side and then on the other.

- This stretch should be started gently and gradually increased.

A2 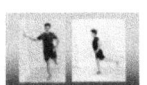 **Swinging Hamstring Stretch**
Sets: 1 Reps: 10
Tempo: Med

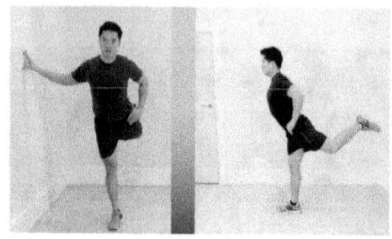 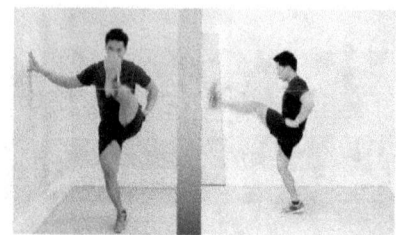

- Stand with feet hip width apart and one hand on a wall to your side.

- Swing your leg forward slightly stretching the back of that leg.

- Swing the same leg back behind your body.

- Repeat the movement gradually increasing the stretch each time.

- Complete all your reps on one side and then on the other.

- This stretch should be started gently and gradually increased.

A3 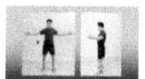 **Swinging Pectoral Stretch**
Sets: 1   Reps: 10
Tempo: Med

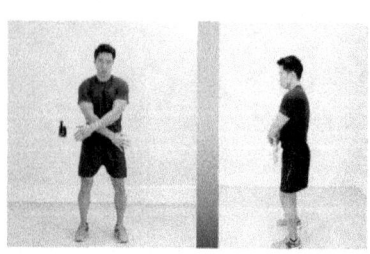 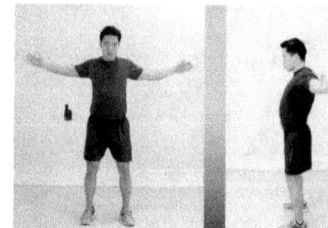

- Stand with your arms out in front of your shoulders and palms facing each other.

- Swing your arms out to the sides and back behind your shoulders to get a stretch in your chest.

- Swing your arms in front of your body before coming back out again.

- Push the stretch a little further with each repetition.

A4 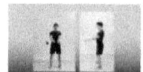 **Arm Circles**
Sets: 1   Reps: 10

Tempo: Med

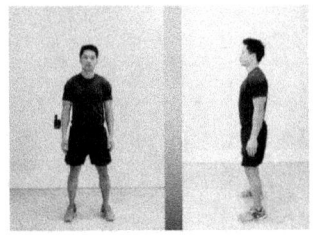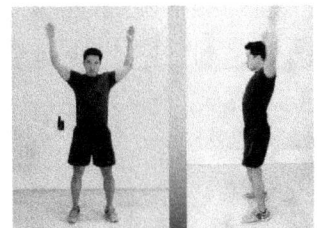

- Stand with feet hip width apart.

- Circle your arms forward and up then back and down.

- Repeat until loose and then change direction.

A5 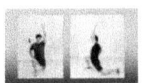 **Lunging Hip Flexor Stretch**
Sets: 1   Reps: 10
Tempo: Med

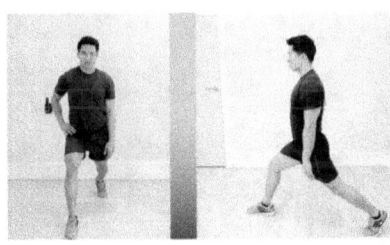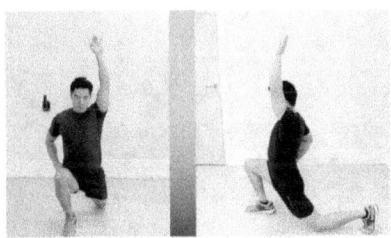

- Push your chest up and draw in your tummy with 30% effort. Step forward approximately 1 ½ times your normal stride length.

- Putting your weight on your front leg, lower yourself forward and down.

- As you come down, push your hips forward, squeeze your bum and raise the arm corresponding with your back leg straight above your shoulder. You should feel a good stretch in front of your hip on the back leg

- Keep your head and chest upright with your hips level and forward facing during the whole movement.

- Repeat the movement on the same leg gradually increasing the stretch.

- Once complete one the first leg repeat the process on the other.

B1 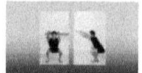 **Metabolic Squat**
Sets: 3   Reps: 12
Tempo: Med   Rest: 30sec
Intensity: 15RM

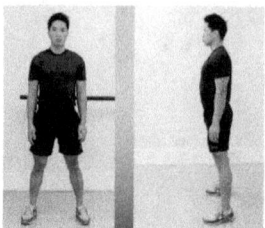 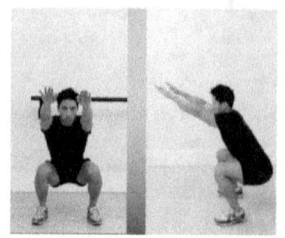

- Stand with your feet a comfortable distance apart.

- Keeping your chest up, bend at your knees then hips to lower your bum down towards the ground behind you.

- Go as low as you can with control, ideally your hips should go below your knees.

- Keeping your heels on the ground, push up into the start position.

C1 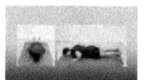 **Press Up Flat**
Sets: 3   Reps: 12
Tempo: Med   Rest: 30sec
Intensity: 15RM

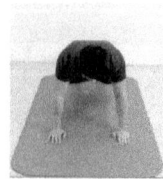 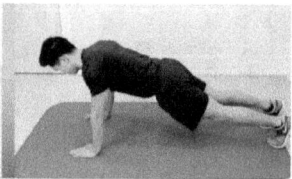 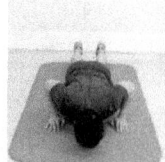 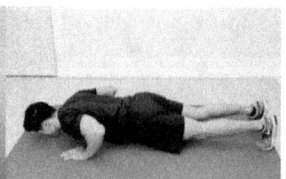

- Come down so that your hands and feet are on the floor.

- Place your hands a little wider than shoulder width apart.

- Position your hips to form a straight line from your heels to your head.

- Gently draw in your tummy using roughly 30% effort.

- Bend your elbows lowering your body toward the ground. Keep your elbows at about 45 degrees from the sides of your body.

- You should come down so that your chest is between your hands.

- Lower until your chest is a small fist away from the ground and then push back up to the start position.

D1 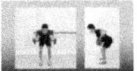   **Bent over Row, Dumbbells - Pronated Grip**
Sets: 3   Reps: 12
Tempo: Med   Rest: 30sec
Intensity: 15RM

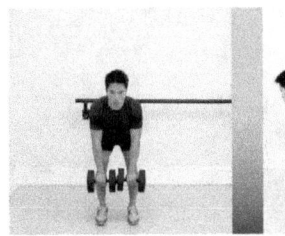 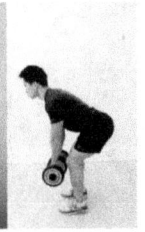 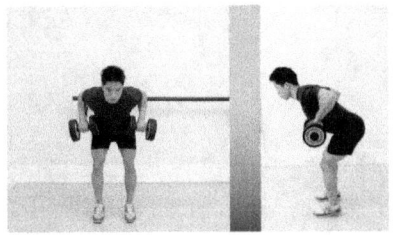

- Stand with feet comfortable and tummy gently drawn in. Lean forward from your hips with a dumbbell in each hand. Your hands should be shoulder width apart and palms facing your body.

- Keeping your shoulders back and down pull the dumbbells in towards the outsides of your bottom ribs.

- Lower the dumbbells under control back down to the starting position.

E1 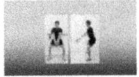   **2 Arm Single Kettlebell Swing**
Sets: 3   Reps: 12
Tempo: Med   Rest: 30sec

Intensity: 15RM

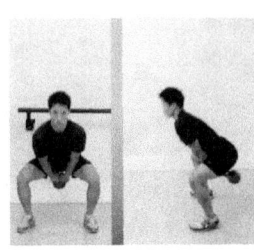 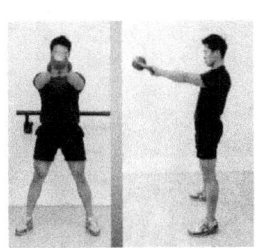

- Stand with your feet wider than shoulder width apart. Take a kettlebell in both hands,

194

lean from your hips to put it on the ground a short distance in front of your body. Push your chest out to straighten your back.

- Keeping your back straight, lift the bell off the ground and swing it gently back between your legs. From this position thrust your hips forward and fully extend your body to power the bell out in front of your body.

- At shoulder height pull the kettlebell back down between your legs ready to thrust forward again.

- Your arms should remain extended throughout the movement.

- To end the movement just take the momentum out of the swing until the kettlebell stops in the bottom position and lower down to the floor.

F1 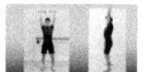 **Standing Shoulder Press - Dumbbells - Pronated Grip**
Sets: 3 Reps: 12
Tempo: Med Rest: 30sec
Intensity: 15RM

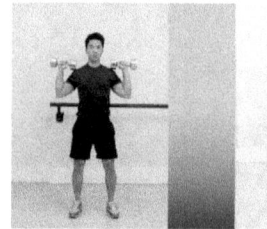 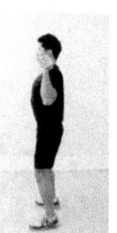 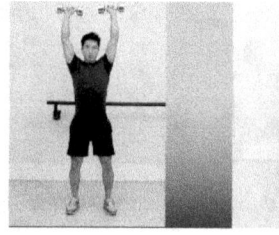 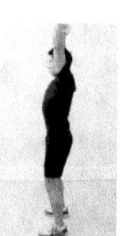

- Stand with your feet hip width apart, tummy gently drawn in with about 30% effort and your shoulders back and down. Lift the dumbbells to shoulder height with your

palms facing forward.

- Keeping your core engaged and body upright push up above your shoulders to a straight arm position.

- Lower under control to the start position.

G1 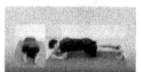 **Plank**
Sets: 3 Reps: 12
Tempo: Med Rest: 30sec
Intensity: 15RM

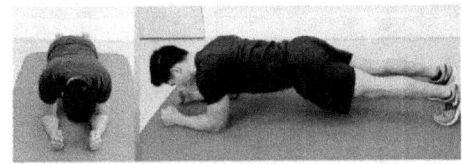

- Come down so that your elbows, feet and hands are touching the floor.

- Engage your core by drawing your tummy in and pelvic floor (the muscle you would use to stop yourself from peeing) up with 30% effort.

- Keep your bum down so your body is flat from your ankles to your head.

- Hold.

H1 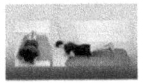 **Foam Roll Quadriceps**
Tempo: 1-2min

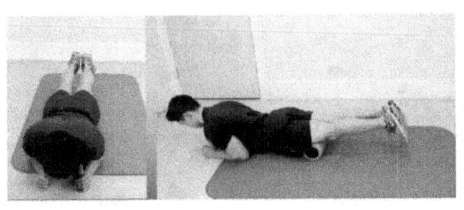 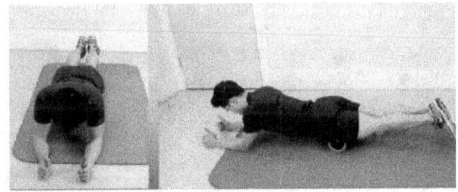

- Lie on your front with the foam roller under your legs placed just above your knees.

- Push from your hands to move your legs slowly over the roller bringing it up towards your hips.

- Roll back down to the starting position.

- To increase the intensity you can do this exercise on one leg at a time.

H2 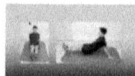 **Foam Roll Hamstrings**
Tempo: 1-2min

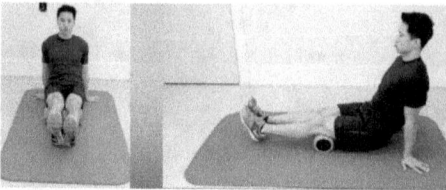 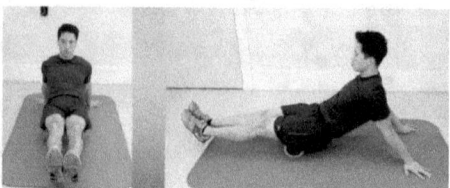

- Sit with the roller under your knees.

- Use your arms to lift your bum and move yourself forward over the roller.

- When the roller gets to your bum, roll back to the start position.

- To increase the intensity you can do this exercise on one leg at a time.

H3 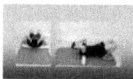 **Foam Roll Thoracic**
Tempo: 1-2min

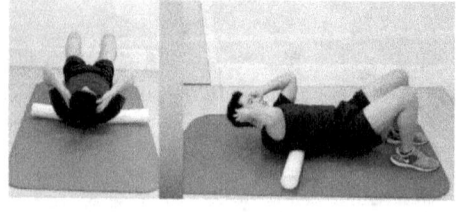 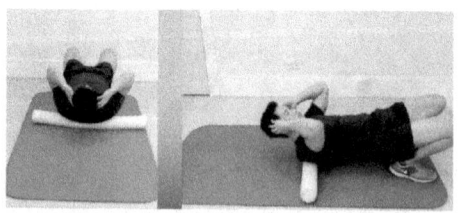

- Lie on your back with a thin roller under the bottom edge of your shoulder blades.

- Move your body across the roller bringing it up towards your shoulders.

- When you get about an inch bellow your shoulders move the other way and bring the roller back into the start position.

Strength & Conditioning

For our last training program, I wanted to include a program structured similarly to the one I used to lose my last 25lbs. Once again, I don't believe in a one-size-fits-all approach to fitness, and I think the program should change and adapt to the needs of the person using it. With that being said my program changed based on my adaptations throughout but this is similar to the program I used.

It starts with a quick power move and then moves to a heavy strength movement. Next, you will see full body moves with isolation movements. This last portion of the full body and isolation are performed in a circuit fashion to help burn calories while still building muscle.

As you can see, it is structured to hit each portion of training. Power, strength, hypertrophy, and endurance. It is an excellent way to all of your muscle fibers and burns fat. Try it and see how it works for you. If you want to explore this type of training further, we have additional programs on our membership site.

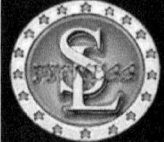
Phase: Phase 1 - Program 1

A1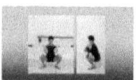

Clean
Sets: 5   Reps: 3
Tempo: Fast   Rest: 2:00
Intensity: 50%1RM

B1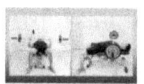

Flat Bench Press - Wide Grip
Sets: 3   Reps: 5
Tempo: 2:1:1   Rest: 3:00
Intensity: 5RM

C1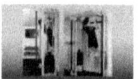

Pull Up - Shoulder Width Grip
Sets: 3   Reps: 10-12
Tempo: 1:1:2   Rest: 1:30
Intensity: 12RM

D1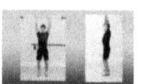

Standing Shoulder Press - Barbell - Shoulder Width Grip
Sets: 3   Reps: 10-12
Tempo: 1:1:2   Rest: 1:30
Intensity: 12RM

E1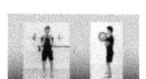

Standing Bicep Curl, EZ Bar - Narrow Grip
Sets: 3   Reps: 12-15
Tempo: 1:1:3   Rest: 1:00
Intensity: 15RM

F1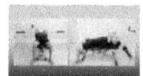

Lying Triceps Extension with Barbell - Narrow Grip
Sets: 3   Reps: 12-15
Tempo: 3:1:1   Rest: 1:00
Intensity: 15RM

G1

Plank
Sets: 3   Reps: 30sec
Tempo: Hold Rest: 1:00

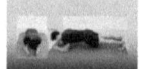

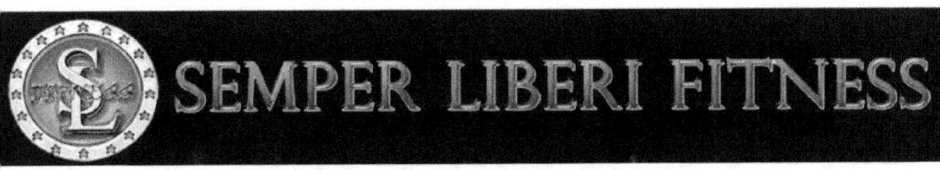

Phase: Phase 1 - Program 1

A1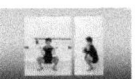

Clean
Sets: 5   Reps: 3
Tempo: Fast   Rest: 2:00
Intensity: 50%1RM

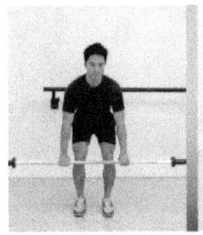 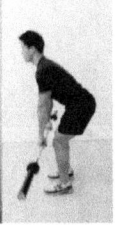 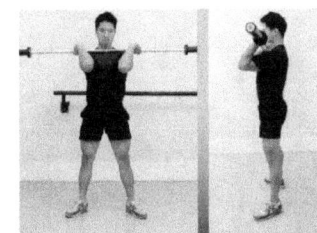

Stand with your feet parallel and shoulder width apart, with weight evenly distributed between both legs and the bar against your shins.

Grip the bar with both hands slightly wider than your legs, using a pronated grip.

Sink your bottom down towards the floor and with a straight back lift the bar up, keeping it against your shins.

As you approach your knees, take them back to allow the bar to clear them, and once cleared, bend the knees under the bar again.

As the bar reaches your upper legs, hit the bar off the top of your thighs, making it travel forward slightly. At this point you need to get under the bar in a wide front squat position, with the bar resting across the front of your shoulders and your elbows high.

Stand upright with the bar to finish the exercise.

B1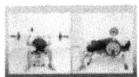

Flat Bench Press - Wide Grip
Sets: 3   Reps: 5
Tempo: 2:1:1   Rest: 3:00
Intensity: 5RM

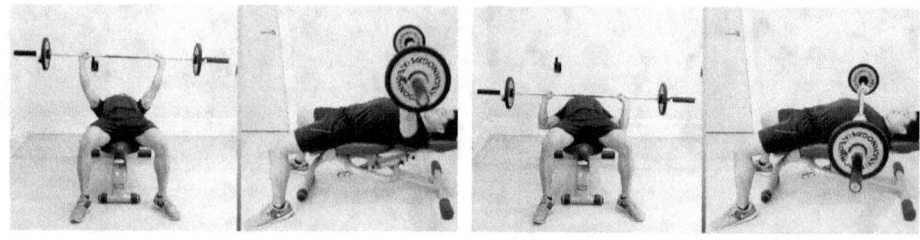

- Lie face up on a bench. Place your hands approximately 1 1/2 times shoulder width apart.

- Take the weight so it sits over your chest.

- Lower the bar under control down towards your chest.

- As the bar touches your chest lift back up to the top position.

- keep your bum, back and head in contact with the bench at all times.

C1 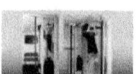 **Pull Up - Shoulder Width Grip**
Sets: 3   Reps: 10-12
Tempo: 1:1:2   Rest: 1:30
Intensity: 12RM

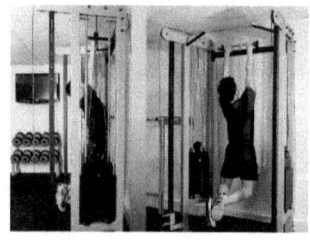 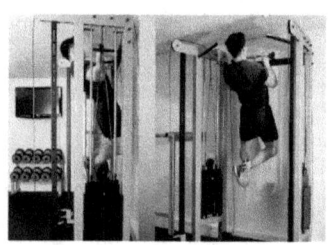

- Stand under the chin up bar at a height where you are able to grip the bar without jumping.

-Take hold of the bar with both hands facing away from you and shoulder width apart. Bring your shoulder blades back towards each other and down towards your bum.

- Pull yourself up to the top position. Your chin should be above your hands and chest pushed out.

- From the top position, lower your self down under control to the bottom.

D1 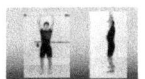 **Standing Shoulder Press - Barbell - Shoulder Width Grip**
Sets: 3   Reps: 10-12
Tempo: 1:1:2   Rest: 1:30
Intensity: 12RM

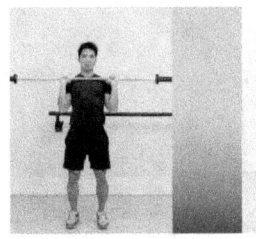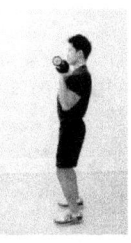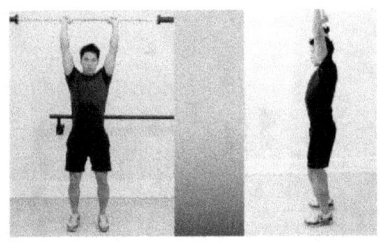

- Stand with your feet hip width apart, tummy gently drawn in with about 30% effort and your shoulders back and down. Take the barbell with a shoulder width grip at shoulder height with your palms facing away from you.

- Keeping your core engaged and body upright push up above your shoulders to a straight arm position.

- Lower under control to the start position.

E1 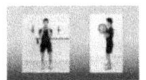 **Standing Bicep Curl, EZ Bar - Narrow Grip**
Sets: 3   Reps: 12-15
Tempo: 1:1:3   Rest: 1:00
Intensity: 15RM

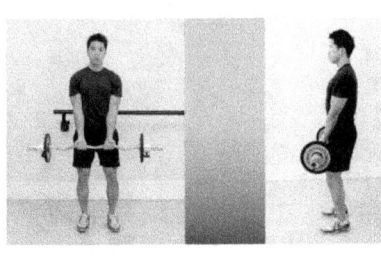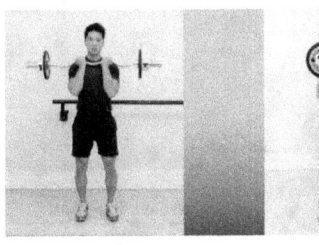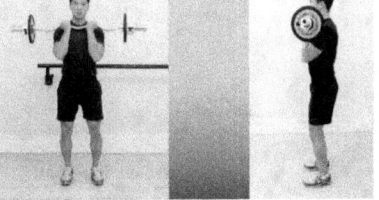

- Stand with feet hip width apart. Take the bar with palms facing away from your body on the inside V of the bar.

202

- Start with elbows straight and your wrists firm.

- Keeping your wrists straight, bend at your elbows until your forearms are in contact with the bulge in your biceps. Don't allow your elbows to come forward in the movement.

- Lower under control back down to the straight arm position.

F1 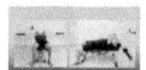 **Lying Triceps Extension with Barbell - Narrow Grip**
Sets: 3   Reps: 12-15
Tempo: 3:1:1   Rest: 1:00
Intensity: 15RM

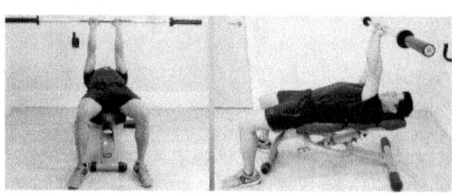 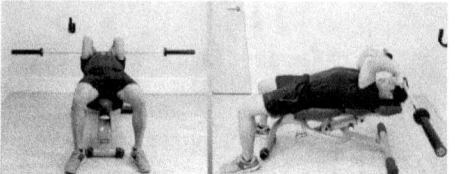

- Lie on the bench facing up. Take the bar with your hands about 2 thumbs apart and your elbows straight.

- Bend at your elbows lowering the bar to just above your forehead.

- Straighten your elbows back into the start position.

G1 **Plank**

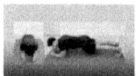 Sets: 3   Reps: 30sec
Tempo: Hold Rest: 1:00

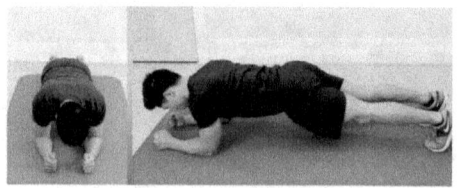

- Come down so that your elbows, feet and hands are touching the floor.

- Engage your core by drawing your tummy in and pelvic floor (the muscle you would use to stop yourself from peeing) up with 30% effort.

- Keep your bum down so your body is flat from your ankles to your head.

- Hold.

Nutrition

I can't write a book about my fitness transformation and try to help you progress in your fitness journey without talking about nutrition. Nutrition is a very important part of your fitness program. Nutrition is much more important than training if you want to achieve your fitness goals.

There is an old saying that nutrition is 80% of your success and training is only 20% (I'm sure this comes from the 80/20 principle in economics) which shows the importance of nutrition in fitness success. While I do think nutrition is a bigger art of fitness success than training, I think there is another variable to consider. I look at the fitness success as being broken up into a pie with 50% being the mindset, goal setting, and belief in success. 40% nutrition, and 10% training.

Old Factors for Success

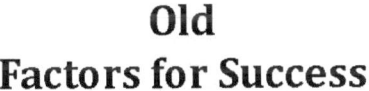

Nutrition 80%

Training 20%

My Factors for Success

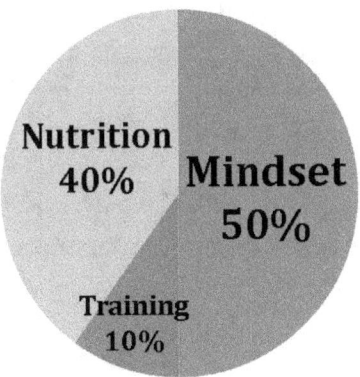

Nutrition 40%

Mindset 50%

Training 10%

You see, the old success model for fitness programs doesn't account for the mental aspect involved in success. I have found in every facet of life that the drive and desire to succeed is the most important factor, and it should be a major focus in any endeavor you begin.

In business, I have also found mindset to be the most important factor and in Think and Grow Rich Napoleon Hill discusses the importance of desire. Finding the driving force and reason you are participating in a program is the most important aspect, and we make that a major part of our coaching program.

Hopefully, I have given you the inspiration and motivation needed to help build the belief that you can be successful and achieve your goals in the first portion of this book. With the second portion you should have the training piece of the pie and be equipped to tackle that aspect of your journey. Now we are going to finish the success equation with nutrition so you have all of the pieces needed for success.

I am not a dietician and I am not authorized to design meal plans. Fitness coaches can give nutritional advice, but as coaches we are limited from strict dietary planning because we are not nutritional professionals.

I wanted to give full disclosure before I give you these nutritional programs and explain that I did not design these and that I am not a nutrition professional.

The included programs were designed by a registered dietitian. I want to ensure that you have all the resources you need to be successful. We design similar programs for our clients and have the ability to make them flexible so that we can include foods they enjoy.

You can't see long term success unless you learn how to use diet and nutrition principles that allow you first to lose weight and then make choices that keep you healthy and let you still enjoy some of the foods you love.

We have included three nutritional programs to get you started based on three different caloric need levels. You will have to calculate your own Basal Metabolic Rate using the included formula or by visiting www.slf.fit/free and using the calculator. Once you have your BMR, you can then select the calorie needs closest to your BMR and adjust accordingly.

You also have access to many recipes, food lists, and a portion guide so you have help building you own healthy meals. This is not a personalized solution like the one we can offer you with our meal planning services, but it will get you a start toward your goal.

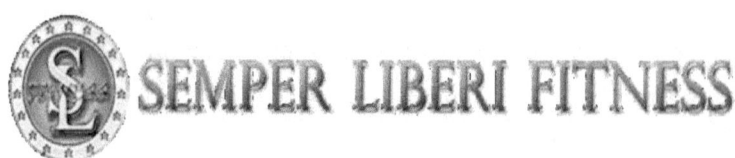

SEMPER LIBERI FITNESS

Use the calculations on the right or visit :

semperliberifitness.com/en/artic les/makeyourownmealplan/

to calculate your BMR.

Once you have your BMR calculations then select the meal plan below that is the closest to your BMR.

Follow the meal plan with the workout plan for the next 14-Days to get the best results.

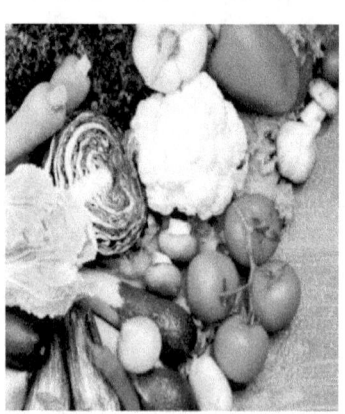

Calculate Basal Metabolic Rate for Women

Women: 655 + (4.35 x weight in pounds) + (4.7 x height in inches) – (4.7 x age in years)

Example 1: You are a 38-year-old woman, who is 5'4" and 142 pounds. First, convert your into inches. 5'4" equals 64 inches. Now include your values into the equation above.

- 655 + (4.35 x 142) + (4.7 x 64) – (4.7 x 38)

- 655 + 617.7 + 300.8 – 178.6 = 1394.9

- **Your BMR = 1394.9**

Example: You are a 28-year-old woman, who is 5'7" and 172 pounds. First, convert your h into inches. 5'4" equals 64 inches. Now include your values into the equation above.

- 655 + (4.35 x 172) + (4.7 x 67) – (4.7 x 28)

- 655 + 748.2 + 314.9 – 131.6 = 1586.5

- **Your BMR = 1586.5**

Calculate Basal Metabolic Rate for Men

Men: 66 + (6.23 x weight in pounds) + (12.7 x height in inches) – (6.8 x age in years)

Example: You are a 40-year-old man, who is 5'9" and 175 pounds. First, convert your heig inches. 5'9" equals 69 inches. Now input your values into the equation above.

- 66 + (6.23 x 175) + (12.7 x 69) – (6.8 x 40)

- 66 + 1090.3 + 876.3 – 272 = 1694.6

- **Your BMR = 1694.6**

Calculate Total Calorie Needs

- **Sedentary** (little or no exercise): BMR x 1.2

- **Lightly active** (easy exercise/sports 1-3 days/week): BMR x 1.375

- **Moderately active** (moderate exercise/sports 3-5 days/week): BMR x 1.55

- **Very active** (hard exercise/sports 6-7 days a week): BMR x 1.725

- **Extremely active** (very hard exercise/sports and physical job): BMR x 1.9

1500 Calorie Meal Plan

Meal Plan
SLF Monthly Meal Plan

Prepared By: James Mullins
Email: semperliberifitness@gmail.com
Created: 10-11-2015

SLF Monthly Plan — Day 1

Day 1

Time	Meal Label	Calories	Meal Items
07:00 am	Breakfast	0	16 fl oz WATER, DRINKING WATER, PURIFIED
		74	1 large EGG, CHICKEN, POACHED
		110	1 cups ORANGE JUICE
		131	1 1/2 cups OAT BRAN, COOKED
Notes:			
Meal Totals:		**Calories: 315**	Carbs: 63g (62%) Protein: 19g (18%) Fat: 9g (20%) Fluid: 36oz
10:00 am	Snack	0	16 fl oz WATER, DRINKING WATER, PURIFIED
		60	1 fruit NECTARINE, RAW
		172	1 cups CHEESE, COTTAGE 1%
Notes:			
Meal Totals:		**Calories: 232**	Carbs: 21g (35%) Protein: 32g (54%) Fat: 3g (11%) Fluid: 28oz
12:00 pm	Lunch	2	1 leaf LETTUCE, COS OR ROMAINE, RAW
		160	2 slice 100% WHOLE WHEAT BREAD
		4	1 oz TOMATO, RAW
		45	1 oz CHICKEN, BROILER, BREAST, MEAT, ROASTED
		5	1 teaspoons MUSTARD, PREPARED, DIJON
		0	16 fl oz WATER, DRINKING WATER, PURIFIED
		80	1 slice CHEDDAR CHEESE, MEDIUM, SLICE
		51	1/2 oz PRETZEL STICKS
Notes:			
Meal Totals:		**Calories: 347**	Carbs: 42g (49%) Protein: 23g (27%) Fat: 9g (24%) Fluid: 20oz
03:00 pm	Snack	0	8 fl oz WATER, DRINKING WATER, PURIFIED
		140	1 bar GRANOLA BAR, CHEWY, HONEY ALMOND FLAX
		91	1 cups MILK, COW'S, NONFAT VIT-D ADDED (SKIM)
Notes:			
Meal Totals:		**Calories: 231**	Carbs: 32g (53%) Protein: 15g (25%) Fat: 6g (22%) Fluid: 16oz
06:00 pm	Dinner	60	1 1/2 teaspoons OLIVE OIL, EXTRA VIRGIN
		0	16 fl oz WATER, DRINKING WATER, PURIFIED
		168	3/4 cups QUINOA, COOKED
		47	2 oz HALIBUT, ATLANTIC & PACIFIC, BAKED OR BROILED
		31	3 oz BRUSSELS SPROUTS, BOILED, NO SALT
Notes:			
Meal Totals:		**Calories: 306**	Carbs: 35g (46%) Protein: 17g (22%) Fat: 11g (32%) Fluid: 20oz

Continued on next page

SLF Monthly Plan — Day 1

Day 1

Time	Meal Label	Calories	Meal Items
08:00 pm	Snack	46	8 large STRAWBERRY, RAW
		0	8 fl oz WATER, DRINKING WATER, PURIFIED
		40	1/4 cups WHIPPED CREAM TOPPING, LIGHT
Notes:			
Meal Totals:		**Calories: 86**	Carbs: 17g (76%) Protein: 1g (4%) Fat: 2g (20%) Fluid: 13oz

		Calories	Carbs	Protein	Fat	Fluid
	Day 1 Totals:	1517	210g (52%)	107g (26%)	40g (22%)	133oz

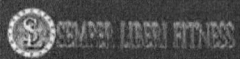
Meal Plan
SLF Monthly Meal Plan

Prepared By: James Mullins
Email: semperliberifitness@gmail.com
Created: 10-11-2015

SLF Monthly Plan   **Day 2**

Day 2

Time	Meal Label	Calories	Meal Items
07:00 am	Breakfast	137	1 1/2 cups MILK, COW'S, NONFAT VIT-D ADDED (SKIM)
		0	16 fl oz WATER, DRINKING WATER, PURIFIED
		155	1 1/2 cups WHEAT CHEX, RTE
Notes:			
Meal Totals:	**Calories: 292**	**Carbs: 52g (68%)**	**Protein: 20g (26%) Fat: 2g (6%) Fluid: 28oz**
10:00 am	Snack	152	1 1/2 tablespoons ALMOND BUTTER, NO SALT
		0	16 fl oz WATER, DRINKING WATER, PURIFIED
		55	1 small APPLE W/SKIN, RAW
Notes:			
Meal Totals:	**Calories: 207**	**Carbs: 20g (36%)**	**Protein: 4g (7%) Fat: 14g (57%) Fluid: 21oz**
12:00 pm	Lunch	90	3 oz ALBACORE TUNA IN WATER, CHUNK WHITE, CANNED, LOWER SODIUM
		2	1 leaf LETTUCE, COS OR ROMAINE, RAW
		75	1 pita BREAD, PITA, WHOLE WHEAT
		0	16 fl oz WATER, DRINKING WATER, PURIFIED
		83	1 cups CARROT, BABY, RAW
		67	2 teaspoons MAYONNAISE, OLIVE OIL, ARTISAN
Notes:			
Meal Totals:	**Calories: 317**	**Carbs: 16g (23%)**	**Protein: 30g (44%) Fat: 10g (33%) Fluid: 21oz**
03:00 pm	Snack	0	16 fl oz WATER, DRINKING WATER, PURIFIED
		140	1 bar GRANOLA BAR, CHEWY, HONEY ALMOND FLAX
		60	1 fruit NECTARINE, RAW
Notes:			
Meal Totals:	**Calories: 200**	**Carbs: 35g (67%)**	**Protein: 6g (11%) Fat: 5g (22%) Fluid: 21oz**
06:00 pm	Dinner	35	1 teaspoons BUTTER
		22	1 cups MUSTARD GREENS, BOILED, DRAINED
		158	6 oz POTATO, BAKED, FLESH & SKIN
		0	16 fl oz WATER, DRINKING WATER, PURIFIED
		62	2 oz BEEF, LOIN, T-BONE STEAK, LEAN, 0 TRIM, BROILED
Notes:			
Meal Totals:	**Calories: 277**	**Carbs: 39g (55%)**	**Protein: 16g (23%) Fat: 7g (22%) Fluid: 28oz**
08:00 pm	Snack	0	8 fl oz WATER, DRINKING WATER, PURIFIED
		90	1 small BANANA, RAW
		127	2/3 cups YOGURT, VANILLA, LOWFAT

SLF Monthly Plan   **Day 2**

Day 2

Time	Meal Label	Calories		Meal Items	
Meal Totals:	**Calories: 217**	**Carbs: 44g (81%)**	**Protein: 8g (15%)**	**Fat: 1g (4%)**	**Fluid: 11oz**
		Calories	Carbs	Protein	Fat	Fluid
Day 2 Totals:		**1510**	**206g (55%)**	**84g (22%)**	**39g (23%)**	**130oz**

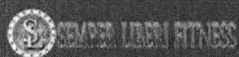
Meal Plan
SLF Monthly Meal Plan

Prepared By: James Mullins
Email: semperliberifitness@gmail.com
Created: 10-11-2015

SLF Monthly Plan

Day 3

Day 3

Time	Meal Label	Calories	Meal Items
07:00 am	Breakfast	60	1 fruit NECTARINE, RAW
		0	16 fl oz WATER, DRINKING WATER, PURIFIED
		80	1 slice 100% WHOLE WHEAT BREAD
		91	1 cups MILK, COW'S, NONFAT VIT-D ADDED (SKIM)
		101	1 tablespoons ALMOND BUTTER, NO SALT

Notes:

| Meal Totals: Calories: 332 | Carbs: 42g (50%) | Protein: 17g (20%) | Fat: 11g (30%) | Fluid: 30oz |

Time	Meal Label	Calories	Meal Items
10:00 am	Snack	0	16 fl oz WATER, DRINKING WATER, PURIFIED
		55	1 small APPLE W/SKIN, RAW
		140	1 bar GRANOLA BAR, CHEWY, HONEY ALMOND FLAX

Notes:

| Meal Totals: Calories: 196 | Carbs: 35g (69%) | Protein: 5g (10%) | Fat: 5g (22%) | Fluid: 20oz |

Time	Meal Label	Calories	Meal Items
12:00 pm	Lunch	185	6 oz BEEF, LOIN, T-BONE STEAK, LEAN, 0 TRIM, BROILED
		0	2 oz TOMATO, RAW
		16	2 cups LETTUCE, COS OR ROMAINE, RAW
		2	1 teaspoons BALSAMIC VINEGAR
		40	1 teaspoons OLIVE OIL, EXTRA VIRGIN
		75	1 roll ROLL, DINNER, WHOLE WHEAT
		2	16 fl oz ICED TEA, UNSWEETENED

Notes:

| Meal Totals: Calories: 328 | Carbs: 19g (24%) | Protein: 30g (37%) | Fat: 14g (39%) | Fluid: 27oz |

Time	Meal Label	Calories	Meal Items
03:00 pm	Snack	76	3/4 oz PRETZEL STICKS
		54	2 tablespoons HUMMUS (SEASONED MASHED CHICKPEA)
		0	16 fl oz WATER, DRINKING WATER, PURIFIED
		62	3/4 cups CARROT, BABY, RAW

Notes:

| Meal Totals: Calories: 192 | Carbs: 33g (70%) | Protein: 3g (9%) | Fat: 3g (21%) | Fluid: 17oz |

Time	Meal Label	Calories	Meal Items
06:00 pm	Dinner	75	1 pita BREAD, PITA, WHOLE WHEAT
		0	16 fl oz WATER, DRINKING WATER, PURIFIED
		18	4 oz SQUASH, SUMMER, CROOKNECK, BOILED, DRAINED
		218	**SAGE & GARLIC ROASTED CHICKEN (TOTALS) (1 Servings)**

Notes:

| Meal Totals: Calories: 311 | Carbs: 22g (28%) | Protein: 31g (39%) | Fat: 12g (34%) | Fluid: 20oz |

Continued on next page...

SLF Monthly Plan

Day 3

Day 3

Time	Meal Label	Calories	Meal Items
08:00 pm	Snack	0	8 fl oz WATER, DRINKING WATER, PURIFIED
		62	1 cups BLACKBERRY, RAW
		95	1/2 cups YOGURT, VANILLA, LOWFAT

Notes:

| Meal Totals: Calories: 157 | Carbs: 30g (71%) | Protein: 8g (19%) | Fat: 2g (11%) | Fluid: 13oz |

	Calories	Carbs	Protein	Fat	Fluid
Day 3 Totals:	1515	172g (46%)	94g (25%)	47g (28%)	127oz

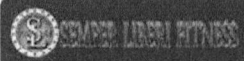
Meal Plan
SLF Monthly Meal Plan

Prepared By: **James Mullins**
Email: **semperliberifitness@gmail.com**
Created: **10-11-2015**

SLF Monthly Plan **Day 4**

Day 4

Time	Meal Label	Calories	Meal Items
07:00 am	Breakfast	55	1/2 cups ORANGE JUICE
		10	2 tablespoons SALSA
		101	1 large EGG, CHICKEN, SCRAMBLED
		170	1 wrap WRAP, 100% WHOLE WHEAT
		0	16 fl oz WATER, DRINKING WATER, PURIFIED

Notes:

Meal Totals:	Calories: 336	Carbs: 43g (52%)	Protein: 13g (16%)	Fat: 12g (33%)	Fluid: 23oz

Time	Meal Label	Calories	Meal Items
10:00 am	Snack	60	1 fruit NECTARINE, RAW
		0	16 fl oz WATER, DRINKING WATER, PURIFIED
		129	3/4 cups CHEESE, COTTAGE 1%

Notes:

Meal Totals:	Calories: 189	Carbs: 19g (40%)	Protein: 24g (51%)	Fat: 7g (9%)	Fluid: 17oz

Time	Meal Label	Calories	Meal Items
12:00 pm	Lunch	75	1 roll ROLL, DINNER, WHOLE WHEAT
		0	16 fl oz WATER, DRINKING WATER, PURIFIED
		109	**SAGE & GARLIC ROASTED CHICKEN (TOTALS) (0.5 Servings)**
		90	1 cups MIXED VEGETABLES, FROZEN

Notes:

Meal Totals:	Calories: 274	Carbs: 33g (49%)	Protein: 19g (28%)	Fat: 7g (23%)	Fluid: 17oz

Time	Meal Label	Calories	Meal Items
03:00 pm	Snack	140	1 bar GRANOLA BAR, CHEWY, HONEY ALMOND FLAX
		0	12 fl oz WATER, DRINKING WATER, PURIFIED
		61	2/3 cups MILK, COW'S, NONFAT VIT-D ADDED (SKIM)

Notes:

Meal Totals:	Calories: 201	Carbs: 28g (55%)	Protein: 12g (23%)	Fat: 5g (22%)	Fluid: 17oz

Time	Meal Label	Calories	Meal Items
06:00 pm	Dinner	108	1/2 cups BROWN RICE, LONG GRAIN, COOKED
		11	1/2 cups MUSTARD GREENS, BOILED, DRAINED
		0	16 fl oz WATER, DRINKING WATER, PURIFIED
		115	2 oz PORK CENTER LOIN, BRAISED, SLO
		78	1/4 cups BEAN, NAVY, CANNED

Notes:

Meal Totals:	Calories: 312	Carbs: 38g (48%)	Protein: 27g (34%)	Fat: 6g (17%)	Fluid: 26oz

Time	Meal Label	Calories	Meal Items
08:00 pm	Snack	0	8 fl oz WATER, DRINKING WATER, PURIFIED
		90	1 small BANANA, RAW
		95	1/2 cups YOGURT, VANILLA, LOWFAT

Notes:

Continued on next page.

SLF Monthly Plan **Day 4**

Day 4

Time	Meal Label	Calories		Meal Items		
	Meal Totals:	Calories: 185	Carbs: 39g (81%)	Protein: 7g (15%)	Fat: 3g (5%)	Fluid: 11oz
		Calories	Carbs	Protein	Fat	Fluid
	Day 4 Totals:	1497	200g (53%)	102g (27%)	33g (20%)	121oz

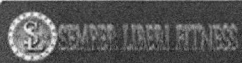
Meal Plan
SLF Monthly Meal Plan

Prepared By: James Mullins
Email: semperliberifitness@gmail.com
Created: 10-11-2015

SLF Monthly Plan   Day 5

Day 5

Time	Meal Label	Calories	Meal Items
07:00 am	Breakfast	155	1 1/2 cups WHEAT CHEX, RTE
		0	16 fl oz WATER, DRINKING WATER, PURIFIED
		137	1 1/2 cups MILK, COW'S, NONFAT VIT D ADDED (SKIM)
Notes:			
	Meal Totals:	Calories: 292	Carbs: 52g (68%) Protein: 20g (26%) Fat: 2g (6%) Fluid: 29oz
10:00 am	Snack	101	1 tablespoons ALMOND BUTTER, NO SALT
		55	1 small APPLE W/SKIN, RAW
		0	16 fl oz WATER, DRINKING WATER, PURIFIED
Notes:			
	Meal Totals:	Calories: 156	Carbs: 18g (45%) Protein: 2g (5%) Fat: 9g (50%) Fluid: 21oz
12:00 pm	Lunch	38	1/2 roll ROLL, DINNER, WHOLE WHEAT
		53	2 oz POTATO, BAKED, FLESH & SKIN
		115	2 oz PORK CENTER LOIN, BRAISED, SLD
		0	16 fl oz WATER, DRINKING WATER, PURIFIED
		2	1 teaspoons BALSAMIC VINEGAR
		16	2 cups LETTUCE, COS OR ROMAINE, RAW
		20	1/2 teaspoons OLIVE OIL, EXTRA VIRGIN
Notes:			
	Meal Totals:	Calories: 244	Carbs: 23g (38%) Protein: 20g (33%) Fat: 8g (30%) Fluid: 25oz
03:00 pm	Snack	101	1 oz PRETZEL STICKS
		83	1 cups CARROT, BABY, RAW
		0	16 fl oz WATER, DRINKING WATER, PURIFIED
		54	2 tablespoons HUMMUS (SEASONED MASHED CHICKPEA)
Notes:			
	Meal Totals:	Calories: 238	Carbs: 29g (75%) Protein: 3g (6%) Fat: 3g (17%) Fluid: 17oz
06:00 pm	Dinner	0	16 fl oz WATER, DRINKING WATER, PURIFIED
		320	**CHOPPED KALE SALAD WITH CHICKEN (TOTALS) (1 Servings)**
		19	1/4 pita BREAD, PITA, WHOLE WHEAT
Notes:			
	Meal Totals:	Calories: 339	Carbs: 19g (23%) Protein: 41g (47%) Fat: 12g (31%) Fluid: 17oz
08:00 pm	Snack	0	8 fl oz WATER, DRINKING WATER, PURIFIED
		90	1 small BANANA, RAW
		140	1 bar GRANOLA BAR, CHEWY, HONEY ALMOND FLAX
Notes:			

Continued on next page...

SLF Monthly Plan   Day 5

Day 5

Time	Meal Label	Calories			Meal Items	
	Meal Totals:	Calories: 230	Carbs: 44g (72%)	Protein: 6g (10%)	Fat: 5g (18%)	Fluid: 11oz
		Calories	Carbs	Protein	Fat	Fluid
	Day 5 Totals:	1499	185g (51%)	92g (25%)	39g (24%)	119oz

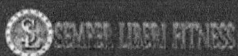
Meal Plan
SLF Monthly Meal Plan

Prepared By: James Mullins
Email: semperliberifitness@gmail.com
Created: 10-11-2015

SLF Monthly Plan

Day 6

Day 6

Time	Meal Label	Calories	Meal Items
07:00 am	Breakfast	90	1 small BANANA, RAW
		0	16 fl oz WATER, DRINKING WATER, PURIFIED
		80	1 slice 100% WHOLE WHEAT BREAD
		101	1 tablespoons ALMOND BUTTER, NO SALT
		91	1 cups MILK, COW'S, NONFAT VIT-D ADDED (SKIM)
Notes:			
	Meal Totals	**Calories: 367**	Carbs: 51g (55%) Protein: 17g (18%) Fat: 11g (27%) Fluid: 28oz
10:00 am	Snack	60	1 fruit NECTARINE, RAW
		0	16 fl oz WATER, DRINKING WATER, PURIFIED
		143	3/4 cups YOGURT, VANILLA, LOWFAT
Notes:			
	Meal Totals	**Calories: 203**	Carbs: 47g (73%) Protein: 9g (18%) Fat: 2g (9%) Fluid: 21oz
12:00 pm	Lunch	2	16 fl oz ICED TEA, UNSWEETENED
		38	1/2 roll ROLL, DINNER, WHOLE WHEAT
		320	**CHOPPED KALE SALAD WITH CHICKEN (TOTALS) (1 Servings)**
Notes:			
	Meal Totals	**Calories: 360**	Carbs: 22g (24%) Protein: 41g (44%) Fat: 13g (32%) Fluid: 18oz
03:00 pm	Snack	55	1 small APPLE W/SKIN, RAW
		140	1 bar GRANOLA BAR, CHEWY, HONEY ALMOND FLAX
		0	16 fl oz WATER, DRINKING WATER, PURIFIED
Notes:			
	Meal Totals	**Calories: 195**	Carbs: 36g (69%) Protein: 5g (10%) Fat: 5g (20%) Fluid: 20oz
06:00 pm	Dinner	162	3/4 cups BROWN RICE, LONG GRAIN, COOKED
		18	4 oz SQUASH, SUMMER, CROOKNECK, BOILED, DRAINED
		35	1 teaspoons BUTTER
		0	16 fl oz WATER, DRINKING WATER, PURIFIED
		92	3 oz SALMON, ATLANTIC, WILD, BAKED OR BROILED
Notes:			
	Meal Totals	**Calories: 307**	Carbs: 38g (50%) Protein: 18g (24%) Fat: 9g (27%) Fluid: 36oz
08:00 pm	Snack	35	6 large STRAWBERRY, RAW
		0	8 fl oz WATER, DRINKING WATER, PURIFIED
		40	1/4 cups WHIPPED CREAM TOPPING, LIGHT
Notes:			
	Meal Totals	**Calories: 75**	Carbs: 14g (72%) Protein: 1g (5%) Fat: 2g (23%) Fluid: 12oz

Continued on next page...

SLF Monthly Plan

Day 6

Day 6

Time	Meal Label	Calories	Meal Items		
		Calories	Carbs	Protein	Fat	Fluid
	Day 6 Totals:	1502	198g (52%)	91g (24%)	42g (25%)	125oz

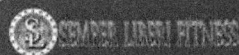
Meal Plan
SLF Monthly Meal Plan

Prepared By: James Mullins
Email: semperliberifitness@gmail.com
Created: 10-11-2015

SLF Monthly Plan Day 7

Day 7

Time	Meal Label	Calories	Meal Items
07:00 am	Breakfast	35	1 teaspoons BUTTER
		110	1 cups ORANGE JUICE
		0	16 fl oz WATER, DRINKING WATER, PURIFIED
		80	1 slice 100% WHOLE GRAIN BREAD
		91	1/4 cups EGG, CHICKEN, SCRAMBLED

Notes:

	Meal Totals:	Calories: 316	Carbs: 44g (52%) Protein: 12g (14%) Fat: 13g (34%) Fluid: 27oz

10:00 am	Snack	51	1/2 oz PRETZEL STICKS
		83	1 cups CARROT, BABY, RAW
		0	16 fl oz WATER, DRINKING WATER, PURIFIED
		54	2 tablespoons HUMMUS (SEASONED MASHED CHICKPEA)

Notes:

	Meal Totals:	Calories: 188	Carbs: 18g (67%) Protein: 2g (7%) Fat: 3g (25%) Fluid: 17oz

12:00 pm	Lunch	2	1 leaf LETTUCE, COS OR ROMAINE, RAW
		4	1 oz TOMATO, RAW
		167	2 oz TURKEY BREAST, ROASTED
		170	1 wrap WRAP, 100% WHOLE WHEAT
		0	16 fl oz WATER, DRINKING WATER, PURIFIED
		5	1 teaspoons MUSTARD, PREPARED, DIJON

Notes:

	Meal Totals:	Calories: 288	Carbs: 29g (41%) Protein: 21g (30%) Fat: 9g (29%) Fluid: 21oz

03:00 pm	Snack	143	3/4 cups YOGURT, VANILLA, LOWFAT
		35	6 large STRAWBERRY, RAW
		0	16 fl oz WATER, DRINKING WATER, PURIFIED

Notes:

	Meal Totals:	Calories: 178	Carbs: 21g (70%) Protein: 9g (20%) Fat: 2g (10%) Fluid: 20oz

06:00 pm	Dinner	90	2 oz CHICKEN, BROILER, BREAST, MEAT, ROASTED
		41	4 oz BRUSSELS SPROUTS, BOILED, NO SALT
		168	3/4 cups QUINOA, COOKED
		0	16 fl oz WATER, DRINKING WATER, PURIFIED

Notes:

	Meal Totals:	Calories: 299	Carbs: 37g (49%) Protein: 28g (37%) Fat: 5g (15%) Fluid: 22oz

08:00 pm	Snack	0	8 fl oz WATER, DRINKING WATER, PURIFIED
		90	1 small BANANA, RAW
		140	1 bar GRANOLA BAR, CHEWY, HONEY ALMOND FLAX

Continued on next page...

SLF Monthly Plan Day 7

Day 7

Time	Meal Label	Calories	Meal Items
Notes:			

	Meal Totals:	Calories: 230	Carbs: 44g (72%) Protein: 6g (10%) Fat: 5g (18%) Fluid: 11oz

		Calories	Carbs	Protein	Fat	Fluid
	Day 7 Totals:	1499	203g (56%)	78g (21%)	37g (23%)	118oz

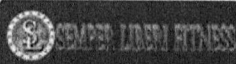 
Meal Plan Shopping List

Category	Quantity	Item
Accompaniments	1/2 cups	Whipped Cream Topping, Light | Cool Whip
	2 tablespoons	Salsa
	2 teaspoons	Mayonnaise, Olive Oil, Artisan | Spectrum
	2 teaspoons	Mustard, Prepared, Dijon | Grey Poupon
Beef	8 oz	Beef, Loin, T-bone Steak, Lean, 0 Trim, Broiled
Beverages	2 1/2 cups	Orange Juice
	6 2/3 cups	Milk, Cow's, Nonfat Vit-d Added (skim)
	32 fl oz	Iced Tea, Unsweetened | Generic
	572 fl oz	Water, Drinking Water, Purified
Bread	1 slice	100% Whole Grain Bread | Healthy Choice
	2 wrap	Wrap, 100% Whole Wheat | Sahara
	2 1/4 pita	Bread, Pita, Whole Wheat
	3 roll	Roll, Dinner, Whole Wheat
	4 slice	100% Whole Wheat Bread | Sara Lee
Cereal and Grain Products	1 1/4 cups	Brown Rice, Long Grain, Cooked
	1 1/2 cups	Oat Bran, Cooked
Cereals, Ready to Eat	3 cups	Wheat Chex, Rte | Ralston
Dairy Products	1/4 cups	Egg, Chicken, Scrambled
	3 1/4 cups	Yogurt, Vanilla, Lowfat | Mountain High
	1 large	Egg, Chicken, Poached
	1 large	Egg, Chicken, Scrambled
	1 slice	Cheddar Cheese, Medium, Slice | Sargento
	1 3/4 cups	Cheese, Cottage 1%
	3 teaspoons	Butter
Fats and Oils	3 teaspoons	Olive Oil, Extra Virgin | Bertolli
Finfish and Shellfish Products	2 oz	Halibut, Atlantic & Pacific, Baked Or Broiled
	3 oz	Albacore Tuna In Water, Chunk White, Canned, Lower Sodium | Chicken of the Sea
	3 oz	Salmon, Atlantic, Wild, Baked Or Broiled
Fruits	1 cups	Blackberry, Raw
	4 small	Apple W/skin, Raw
	5 fruit	Nectarine, Raw
	5 small	Banana, Raw
	20 large	Strawberry, Raw
Ingredients	2 teaspoons	Balsamic Vinegar | Spectrum
Legumes	1/4 cups	Bean, Navy, Canned

Continued on next page...

Meal Plan Shopping List

Category	Quantity	Item
	6 tablespoons	Hummus (seasoned Mashed Chickpea)
Nuts and Seeds	4 1/2 tablespoons	Almond Butter, No Salt
Pork	4 oz	Pork Center Loin, Braised, Slo
Poultry	2 oz	Turkey Breast, Roasted
	3 oz	Chicken, Broiler, Breast, Meat, Roasted
Side Dishes	1 1/2 cups	Quinoa, Cooked
	1 cups	Mixed Vegetables, Frozen	Cascadian Farm
Snacks	2 3/4 oz	Pretzel, Sticks	Rold Gold
	7 bar	Granola Bar, Chewy, Honey Almond Flax	Kashi
Vegetables	1 1/2 cups	Mustard Greens, Boiled, Drained
	2 oz	Potato, Baked, Flesh & Skin
	3 leaf	Lettuce, Cos Or Romaine, Raw
	3 3/4 cups	Carrot, Baby, Raw
	4 cups	Lettuce, Cos Or Romaine, Raw
	4 oz	Tomato, Raw
	6 oz	Potato, Baked, Flesh & Skin
	7 oz	Brussels Sprouts, Boiled, No Salt
	8 oz	Squash, Summer, Crookneck, Boiled, Drained

Recipe Shopping List

Category	Quantity	Item
Beverages	2 tablespoons	Lemon Juice
Fats and Oils	4 tablespoons	Olive Oil
Fruits	1 teaspoons	Lemon Peel, Raw
Ingredients	1/4 teaspoons	Salt, Sea
Poultry	8 oz	Chicken Breast, Boneless, Roasted, Meat Only
	16 oz	Chicken, Breast W/o Skin, Raw
Spices	1 tablespoons	Garlic Powder
	1 tablespoons	Sage, Ground
	2 dash	Pepper, Black, Ground
Vegetables	4 cups	Kale, Raw

1750 Calorie Meal Plan

Day 1

Time	Meal Label	Calories	Meal Items
07:00 am	Breakfast	135	1 muffin ENGLISH MUFFIN, WHOLE WHEAT, TOASTED
		147	2 large EGG, CHICKEN, POACHED
		0	16 fl oz WATER, DRINKING WATER, PURIFIED
		110	22 fl oz ALMOND BEVERAGE, VANILLA UNSWEETENED, NONDAIRY

Notes:

Meal Totals:	Calories: 392	Carbs: 44g (29%)	Protein: 22g (18%)	Fat: 35g (53%)	Fluid: 81oz

Time	Meal Label	Calories	Meal Items
10:00 am	Snack	120	2 fruit NECTARINE, RAW
		75	1/4 cups YOGURT, GREEK-STYLE
		0	16 fl oz WATER, DRINKING WATER, PURIFIED

Notes:

Meal Totals:	Calories: 195	Carbs: 41g (38%)	Protein: 12g (11%)	Fat: 24g (50%)	Fluid: 25oz

Time	Meal Label	Calories	Meal Items
12:00 pm	Lunch	101	1 oz PRETZEL STICKS
		2	1 leaf LETTUCE, COS OR ROMAINE, RAW
		80	1 slice CHEDDAR CHEESE, MEDIUM, SLICE
		160	2 slice 100% WHOLE WHEAT BREAD
		4	1 oz TOMATO, RAW
		45	1 oz CHICKEN, BROILER, BREAST, MEAT, ROASTED
		5	1 teaspoons MUSTARD, PREPARED, DIJON
		0	16 fl oz WATER, DRINKING WATER, PURIFIED

Notes:

Meal Totals:	Calories: 397	Carbs: 53g (54%)	Protein: 24g (25%)	Fat: 9g (21%)	Fluid: 20oz

Time	Meal Label	Calories	Meal Items
03:00 pm	Snack	91	1 cups MILK, COW'S, NONFAT VIT D ADDED (SKIM)
		138	2 1/2 tablespoons BROWN RICE CAKE, CORN
		0	8 fl oz WATER, DRINKING WATER, PURIFIED

Notes:

Meal Totals:	Calories: 229	Carbs: 295g (82%)	Protein: 39g (11%)	Fat: 12g (7%)	Fluid: 17oz

Time	Meal Label	Calories	Meal Items
06:00 pm	Dinner	224	1 cups QUINOA, COOKED
		0	16 fl oz WATER, DRINKING WATER, PURIFIED
		60	1 1/2 teaspoons OLIVE OIL, EXTRA VIRGIN
		46	3/4 oz SALMON, SOCKEYE, BAKED OR BROILED
		31	3 oz BRUSSELS SPROUTS, BOILED, NO SALT

Notes:

Meal Totals:	Calories: 361	Carbs: 45g (17%)	Protein: 106g (41%)	Fat: 49g (42%)	Fluid: 27oz

Meal Plan
SLF Plan

Day 1

Time	Meal Label	Calories	Meal Items
08:00 pm	Snack	40	2 tablespoons APPLE BUTTER
		46	8 large STRAWBERRY, RAW
		75	1/4 cups YOGURT, GREEK-STYLE
		0	8 fl oz WATER, DRINKING WATER, PURIFIED

Notes:

Meal Totals:	Calories: 161	Carbs: 27g (30%)	Protein: 10g (11%)	Fat: 23g (58%)	Fluid: 13oz

	Calories	Carbs	Protein	Fat	Fluid
Day 1 Totals:	1735	505g (47%)	218g (20%)	152g (32%)	183oz

Day 2

Time	Meal Label	Calories	Meal Items
07:00 am	Breakfast	74 160 0 137	1 large EGG, CHICKEN, POACHED 2 slice 100% WHOLE GRAIN BREAD 16 fl oz WATER, DRINKING WATER, PURIFIED 1 1/2 cups MILK, COW'S, NONFAT VIT-D ADDED (SKIM)
Notes:			
Meal Totals:	**Calories: 371**	**Carbs: 34g (45%)**	**Protein: 25g (33%)** **Fat: 7g (21%)** **Fluid: 29oz**
10:00 am	Snack	177 0 55	1 3/4 tablespoons ALMOND BUTTER, NO SALT 16 fl oz WATER, DRINKING WATER, PURIFIED 1 small APPLE W/SKIN, RAW
Notes:			
Meal Totals:	**Calories: 232**	**Carbs: 21g (33%)**	**Protein: 4g (6%)** **Fat: 17g (60%)** **Fluid: 21oz**
12:00 pm	Lunch	151 90 67 83 0 2	2 pita BREAD, PITA, WHOLE WHEAT 3 oz ALBACORE TUNA IN WATER, CHUNK WHITE, CANNED, LOWER SODIUM 2 teaspoons MAYONNAISE, OLIVE OIL, ARTISAN 1 cups CARROT, BABY, RAW 16 fl oz WATER, DRINKING WATER, PURIFIED 1 leaf LETTUCE, COS OR ROMAINE, RAW
Notes:			
Meal Totals:	**Calories: 393**	**Carbs: 31g (36%)**	**Protein: 33g (38%)** **Fat: 10g (26%)** **Fluid: 21oz**
03:00 pm	Snack	60 138 0	1 fruit NECTARINE, RAW 2 1/2 tablespoons BROWN RICE CAKE, CORN 16 fl oz WATER, DRINKING WATER, PURIFIED
Notes:			
Meal Totals:	**Calories: 198**	**Carbs: 29g (84%)**	**Protein: 3g (8%)** **Fat: 1g (7%)** **Fluid: 22oz**
06:00 pm	Dinner	62 0 15 35 75 132	2 oz BEEF, LOIN, T-BONE STEAK, LEAN, 0 TRIM, BROILED 16 fl oz WATER, DRINKING WATER, PURIFIED 1/4 cups SPINACH, CHOPPED, FROZEN 1 teaspoons BUTTER 1 roll ROLL, DINNER, WHOLE WHEAT 3/4 cups SWEET POTATO, BAKED, NO SALT
Notes:			
Meal Totals:	**Calories: 319**	**Carbs: 36g (43%)**	**Protein: 15g (17%)** **Fat: 8g (20%)** **Fluid: 24oz**

Continued on next page...

Day 2

Time	Meal Label	Calories	Meal Items
08:00 pm	Snack	133 90 0	1 1/4 cups YOGURT, PLAIN, NONFAT 1 small BANANA, RAW 8 fl oz WATER, DRINKING WATER, PURIFIED
Notes:			
Meal Totals:	**Calories: 223**	**Carbs: 107g (69%)**	**Protein: 49g (31%)** **Fat: 0g (0%)** **Fluid: 11oz**

	Calories	Carbs	Protein	Fat	Fluid
Day 2 Totals:	1736	547g (67%)	156g (19%)	53g (15%)	128oz

Day 3

Time	Meal Label	Calories	Meal Items
07:00 am	Breakfast	91 0 60 160 101	1 cups MILK, COW'S, NONFAT VIT-D ADDED (SKIM) 16 fl oz WATER, DRINKING WATER, PURIFIED 1 fruit NECTARINE, RAW 2 slice 100% WHOLE WHEAT BREAD 1 tablespoons ALMOND BUTTER, NO SALT
Notes:			
	Meal Totals:	Calories: 412	Carbs: 56g (54%) Protein: 21g (20%) Fat: 12g (26%) Fluid: 30oz
10:00 am	Snack	0 55 138	16 fl oz WATER, DRINKING WATER, PURIFIED 1 small APPLE W/SKIN, RAW 2 1/2 tablespoons BROWN RICE CAKE, CORN
Notes:			
	Meal Totals:	Calories: 193	Carbs: 299g (85%) Protein: 29g (8%) Fat: 11g (7%) Fluid: 21oz
12:00 pm	Lunch	112 2 75 40 2 92 16 8	1/2 cups QUINOA, COOKED 16 fl oz ICED TEA, UNSWEETENED 1 roll ROLL, DINNER, WHOLE WHEAT 1 teaspoons OLIVE OIL, EXTRA VIRGIN 1 teaspoons BALSAMIC VINEGAR 3 oz BEEF, LOIN, T-BONE STEAK, LEAN, 0 TRIM, BROILED 2 cups LETTUCE, COS OR ROMAINE, RAW 2 oz TOMATO, RAW
Notes:			
	Meal Totals:	Calories: 347	Carbs: 39g (45%) Protein: 21g (24%) Fat: 12g (31%) Fluid: 26oz
03:00 pm	Snack	101 83 54 0	1 oz PRETZEL, STICKS 1 cups CARROT, BABY, RAW 2 tablespoons HUMMUS (SEASONED MASHED CHICKPEA) 16 fl oz WATER, DRINKING WATER, PURIFIED
Notes:			
	Meal Totals:	Calories: 238	Carbs: 79g (75%) Protein: 3g (8%) Fat: 3g (17%) Fluid: 17oz
06:00 pm	Dinner	75 0 36 218	1 pita BREAD, PITA, WHOLE WHEAT 16 fl oz WATER, DRINKING WATER, PURIFIED 8 oz SQUASH, SUMMER, CROOKNECK, BOILED, DRAINED **SAGE & GARLIC ROASTED CHICKEN (TOTALS) (1 Servings)**
Notes:			
	Meal Totals:	Calories: 329	Carbs: 26g (30%) Protein: 32g (37%) Fat: 13g (34%) Fluid: 23oz

Continued on next page...

Day 3

Time	Meal Label	Calories	Meal Items
08:00 pm	Snack	133 93 0	1 1/4 cups YOGURT, PLAIN, NONFAT 1 1/2 cups BLACKBERRY, RAW 8 fl oz WATER, DRINKING WATER, PURIFIED
Notes:			
	Meal Totals:	Calories: 226	Carbs: 105g (66%) Protein: 51g (32%) Fat: 1g (1%) Fluid: 15oz

		Calories	Carbs	Protein	Fat	Fluid
	Day 3 Totals:	1745	554g (67%)	157g (19%)	52g (14%)	132oz

Day 4

Time	Meal Label	Calories	Meal Items
07:00 am	Breakfast	110	22 fl oz ALMOND BEVERAGE, VANILLA UNSWEETENED, NONDAIRY
		0	16 fl oz WATER, DRINKING WATER, PURIFIED
		101	1 large EGG, CHICKEN, SCRAMBLED
		170	1 wrap WRAP, 100% WHOLE WHEAT
		10	2 tablespoons SALSA

Notes:

| | Meal Totals: | Calories: 391 | Carbs: 46g (31%) | Protein: 20g (14%) | Fat: 36g (55%) | Fluid: 80oz |

10:00 am	Snack	129	3/4 cups CHEESE, COTTAGE 1%
		60	1 fruit NECTARINE, RAW
		0	16 fl oz WATER, DRINKING WATER, PURIFIED

Notes:

| | Meal Totals: | Calories: 189 | Carbs: 19g (40%) | Protein: 24g (51%) | Fat: 2g (9%) | Fluid: 27oz |

12:00 pm	Lunch	90	1 cups MIXED VEGETABLES, FROZEN
		75	1 roll ROLL, DINNER, WHOLE WHEAT
		218	**SAGE & GARLIC ROASTED CHICKEN (TOTALS) (1 Servings)**
		0	16 fl oz WATER, DRINKING WATER, PURIFIED

Notes:

| | Meal Totals: | Calories: 383 | Carbs: 34g (37%) | Protein: 32g (34%) | Fat: 12g (29%) | Fluid: 17oz |

03:00 pm	Snack	46	1/2 oz RAISIN
		0	12 fl oz WATER, DRINKING WATER, PURIFIED
		138	2 1/2 tablespoons BROWN RICE CAKE, CORN
		46	1/2 cups MILK, COW'S, NONFAT VIT-D ADDED (SKIM)

Notes:

| | Meal Totals: | Calories: 230 | Carbs: 299g (83%) | Protein: 35g (10%) | Fat: 11g (7%) | Fluid: 18oz |

06:00 pm	Dinner	156	1/2 cups BEAN, NAVY, CANNED
		108	1/2 cups BROWN RICE, LONG GRAIN, COOKED
		115	2 oz PORK CENTER LOIN, BRAISED, SLO
		17	3/4 cups MUSTARD GREENS, BOILED, DRAINED
		0	16 fl oz WATER, DRINKING WATER, PURIFIED

Notes:

| | Meal Totals: | Calories: 396 | Carbs: 57g (52%) | Protein: 33g (33%) | Fat: 7g (16%) | Fluid: 29oz |

09:00 pm	Snack	0	8 fl oz WATER, DRINKING WATER, PURIFIED
		90	1 small BANANA, RAW
		80	1/4 cups CHEDDAR CHEESE, MILD, SHREDDED, REDUCED FAT

Continued on next page...

Meal Plan
SLF Plan

Day 4

Time	Meal Label	Calories	Meal Items

Notes:

| | Meal Totals: | Calories: 170 | Carbs: 23g (75%) | Protein: 3g (10%) | Fat: 2g (15%) | Fluid: 11oz |

		Calories	Carbs	Protein	Fat	Fluid
	Day 4 Totals:	1759	473g (61%)	147g (19%)	70g (20%)	182oz

Day 5

Time	Meal Label	Calories	Meal Items
07:00 am	Breakfast	52 125 137 0	1 oz BACON, CANADIAN-STYLE, GRILLED 1/2 bagel 100% WHOLE WHEAT BAGEL 1 1/2 cups MILK, COW'S, NONFAT VIT-D ADDED (SKIM) 16 fl oz WATER, DRINKING WATER, PURIFIED
Notes:			
	Meal Totals:	**Calories: 314**	**Carbs: 65g (59%) Protein: 33g (30%) Fat: 5g (10%) Fluid: 28oz**
10:00 am	Snack	152 0 55	1 1/2 tablespoons ALMOND BUTTER, NO SALT 16 fl oz WATER, DRINKING WATER, PURIFIED 1 small APPLE W/SKIN, RAW
Notes:			
	Meal Totals:	**Calories: 207**	**Carbs: 20g (36%) Protein: 4g (7%) Fat: 14g (57%) Fluid: 21oz**
12:00 pm	Lunch	88 20 16 2 115 0 75	1/2 cups SWEET POTATO, BAKED, NO SALT 1/2 teaspoons OLIVE OIL, EXTRA VIRGIN 2 cups LETTUCE, COS OR ROMAINE, RAW 1 teaspoons BALSAMIC VINEGAR 2 oz PORK CENTER LOIN, BRAISED, SLD 16 fl oz WATER, DRINKING WATER, PURIFIED 1 roll ROLL, DINNER, WHOLE WHEAT
Notes:			
	Meal Totals:	**Calories: 316**	**Carbs: 59g (59%) Protein: 23g (23%) Fat: 8g (18%) Fluid: 28oz**
03:00 pm	Snack	83 0 101 54	1 cups CARROT, BABY, RAW 16 fl oz WATER, DRINKING WATER, PURIFIED 1 oz PRETZEL, STICKS 2 tablespoons HUMMUS (SEASONED MASHED CHICKPEA)
Notes:			
	Meal Totals:	**Calories: 238**	**Carbs: 29g (75%) Protein: 3g (8%) Fat: 3g (17%) Fluid: 17oz**
06:00 pm	Dinner	320 38 0	CHOPPED KALE SALAD WITH CHICKEN (TOTALS) (1 Servings) 1/2 pita BREAD, PITA, WHOLE WHEAT 16 fl oz WATER, DRINKING WATER, PURIFIED
Notes:			
	Meal Totals:	**Calories: 358**	**Carbs: 23g (25%) Protein: 41g (45%) Fat: 12g (30%) Fluid: 17oz**

Continued on next page...

Day 5

Time	Meal Label	Calories	Meal Items
08:00 pm	Snack	69 90 0 90	1 1/4 tablespoons BROWN RICE CAKE, CORN 2 tablespoons CHEDDAR CHEESE, SHARP, REDUCED FAT 8 fl oz WATER, DRINKING WATER, PURIFIED 1 small BANANA, RAW
Notes:			
	Meal Totals:	**Calories: 249**	**Carbs: 308g (80%) Protein: 37g (10%) Fat: 17g (10%) Fluid: 12oz**

		Calories	Carbs	Protein	Fat	Fluid
	Day 5 Totals:	**1682**	**504g (65%)**	**141g (18%)**	**59g (17%)**	**123oz**

Day 6

Time	Meal Label	Calories	Meal Items
07:00 am	Breakfast	0 101 90 160 46	16 fl oz WATER, DRINKING WATER, PURIFIED 1 tablespoons ALMOND BUTTER, NO SALT 1 small BANANA, RAW 2 slice 100% WHOLE WHEAT BREAD 1/2 cups MILK, COW'S, NONFAT VIT-D ADDED (SKIM)
Notes:			
	Meal Totals:	**Calories: 397**	**Carbs: 59g (59%) Protein: 16g (16%) Fat: 11g (25%) Fluid: 24oz**
10:00 am	Snack	60 0 220	1 fruit NECTARINE, RAW 16 fl oz WATER, DRINKING WATER, PURIFIED 1/2 cups CHEDDAR CHEESE, DOUBLE, SHREDDED
Notes:			
	Meal Totals:	**Calories: 280**	**Carbs: 14g (65%) Protein: 3g (14%) Fat: 2g (21%) Fluid: 21oz**
12:00 pm	Lunch	2 320 75	16 fl oz ICED TEA, UNSWEETENED **CHOPPED KALE SALAD WITH CHICKEN (TOTALS) (1 Servings)** 1 roll ROLL, DINNER, WHOLE WHEAT
Notes:			
	Meal Totals:	**Calories: 397**	**Carbs: 29g (29%) Protein: 42g (42%) Fat: 13g (29%) Fluid: 18oz**
03:00 pm	Snack	138 55 0	2 1/2 tablespoons BROWN RICE CAKE, CORN 1 small APPLE W/SKIN, RAW 16 fl oz WATER, DRINKING WATER, PURIFIED
Notes:			
	Meal Totals:	**Calories: 193**	**Carbs: 39g (85%) Protein: 2g (8%) Fat: 1g (7%) Fluid: 21oz**
06:00 pm	Dinner	18 62 0 35 216	4 oz SQUASH, SUMMER, CROOKNECK, BOILED, DRAINED 2 oz SALMON, ATLANTIC, WILD, BAKED OR BROILED 16 fl oz WATER, DRINKING WATER, PURIFIED 1 teaspoons BUTTER 1 cups BROWN RICE, LONG GRAIN, COOKED
Notes:			
	Meal Totals:	**Calories: 331**	**Carbs: 49g (58%) Protein: 15g (18%) Fat: 9g (24%) Fluid: 27oz**
08:00 pm	Snack	80 56 0 46	3/4 cups YOGURT, PLAIN, NONFAT 1 tablespoons CEREAL, RTE, GRANOLA, LOWFAT ORIGINAL 8 fl oz WATER, DRINKING WATER, PURIFIED 8 large STRAWBERRY, RAW

Continued on next page...

Day 6

Time	Meal Label	Calories	Meal Items		
Notes:					
	Meal Totals:	**Calories: 182**	**Carbs: 106g (67%) Protein: 50g (32%) Fat: 1g (1%) Fluid: 14oz**		
		Calories	Carbs	Protein	Fat	Fluid
	Day 6 Totals:	**1780**	**556g (68%)**	**155g (19%)**	**47g (13%)**	**125oz**

Day 7

Time	Meal Label	Calories	Meal Items
07:00 am	Breakfast	126	1/4 cups TORTILLA, CORN, NO ADDED SALT, RTC
		75	1 1/2 tablespoons AMERICAN CHEESE
		35	1 teaspoons BUTTER
		0	16 fl oz WATER, DRINKING WATER, PURIFIED
		110	22 fl oz ALMOND BEVERAGE, VANILLA, UNSWEETENED, NONDAIRY

Notes:

| | Meal Totals: | Calories: 346 | Carbs: 30g (23%) | Protein: 16g (12%) | Fat: 38g (65%) | Fluid: 79oz |

Time	Meal Label	Calories	Meal Items
10:00 am	Snack	51	1/2 oz PRETZEL STICKS
		0	16 fl oz WATER, DRINKING WATER, PURIFIED
		79	4 1/2 tablespoons HUMMUS, ORIGINAL
		83	1 cups CARROT, BABY, RAW

Notes:

| | Meal Totals: | Calories: 213 | Carbs: 20g (67%) | Protein: 3g (10%) | Fat: 3g (23%) | Fluid: 16oz |

Time	Meal Label	Calories	Meal Items
12:00 pm	Lunch	3	2 leaf LETTUCE, COS OR ROMAINE, RAW
		8	2 oz TOMATO, RAW
		0	16 fl oz WATER, DRINKING WATER, PURIFIED
		170	1 wrap WRAP, 100% WHOLE WHEAT
		123	4 oz BEEF, LOIN, T-BONE STEAK, LEAN, 0 TRIM, BROILED
		67	2 teaspoons MAYONNAISE, OLIVE OIL, ARTISAN

Notes:

| | Meal Totals: | Calories: 371 | Carbs: 29g (32%) | Protein: 23g (25%) | Fat: 17g (42%) | Fluid: 21oz |

Time	Meal Label	Calories	Meal Items
03:00 pm	Snack	56	1 tablespoons CEREAL, RTE, GRANOLA, LOWFAT-ORIGINAL
		146	3 1/4 tablespoons CHEDDAR CHEESE, SHARP, REDUCED FAT
		0	16 fl oz WATER, DRINKING WATER, PURIFIED
		35	6 large STRAWBERRY, RAW

Notes:

| | Meal Totals: | Calories: 237 | Carbs: 20g (45%) | Protein: 9g (20%) | Fat: 7g (35%) | Fluid: 21oz |

Time	Meal Label	Calories	Meal Items
06:00 pm	Dinner	224	1 cups QUINOA, COOKED
		90	2 oz CHICKEN, BROILER, BREAST, MEAT, ROASTED
		0	16 fl oz WATER, DRINKING WATER, PURIFIED
		41	4 oz BRUSSELS SPROUTS, BOILED, NO SALT

Notes:

| | Meal Totals: | Calories: 355 | Carbs: 47g (52%) | Protein: 30g (33%) | Fat: 6g (15%) | Fluid: 22oz |

Continued on next page...

Day 7

Time	Meal Label	Calories	Meal Items
08:00 pm	Snack	0	8 fl oz WATER, DRINKING WATER, PURIFIED
		90	1 small BANANA, RAW
		138	2 1/2 tablespoons BROWN RICE CAKE, CORN

Notes:

| | Meal Totals: | Calories: 228 | Carbs: 307g (85%) | Protein: 30g (8%) | Fat: 11g (7%) | Fluid: 12oz |

		Calories	Carbs	Protein	Fat	Fluid
	Day 7 Totals:	1750	453g (61%)	111g (15%)	82g (25%)	171oz

Sage & Garlic Roasted Chicken (totals) (serves 4)

Ingredients

- 1 tablespoons Garlic Powder
- 1 tablespoons Sage, Ground
- 3 tablespoons Olive Oil
- 2 dash Pepper, Black, Ground
- 16 oz Chicken, Breast W/o Skin, Raw

Instructions

Preheat oven to 375. Wash chicken inside and out, pat dry with paper towels. In a small bowl, whisk together sage, oil, garlic and pepper. Rub this mixture under the skin of the breast and on the skin all over the chicken. Place chicken, breast side down, on lightly greased pan. Roast for 30 minutes, then turn chicken breast side up and continue roasting until internal temperature reaches 180.

Chopped Kale Salad with Chicken (totals) (serves 2)

Ingredients

- 4 cups Kale, Raw
- 1 teaspoons Lemon Peel, Raw
- 8 oz Chicken Breast, Boneless, Roasted, Meat Only
- 1 tablespoons Olive Oil
- 1/4 teaspoons Salt, Sea
- 2 tablespoons Lemon Juice

Instructions

1. Combine olive oil, lemon juice, lemon zest, salt, and pepper in small bowl.

2. Pour over chopped kale and toss.

3. Divide kale into 2 bowls.

4. Top each bowl of kale with 4 oz of roasted chicken breast.

Meal Plan Shopping List

Category	Quantity	Item
Accompaniments	1 teaspoons	Mustard, Prepared, Dijon | Grey Poupon
	2 tablespoons	Apple Butter | Eden Foods
	2 tablespoons	Salsa
	4 teaspoons	Mayonnaise, Olive Oil, Artisan | Spectrum
Beef	9 oz	Beef, Loin, T-bone Steak, Lean, 0 Trim, Broiled
Beverages	6 cups	Milk, Cow's, Nonfat Vit d Added (skim)
	32 fl oz	Iced Tea, Unsweetened | Generic
	66 fl oz	Almond Beverage, Vanilla Unsweetened, Nondairy | Blue Diamond Almond Breeze
	572 fl oz	Water, Drinking Water, Purified
Bread	1/4 cups	Tortilla, Corn, No Added Salt, Rtc
	1/2 bagel	100% Whole Wheat Bagel | Pepperidge Farm
	1 muffin	English Muffin, Whole Wheat, Toasted
	2 slice	100% Whole Grain Bread | Healthy Choice
	2 wrap	Wrap, 100% Whole Wheat | Sahara
	3 1/2 pita	Bread, Pita, Whole Wheat
	5 roll	Roll, Dinner, Whole Wheat
	6 slice	100% Whole Wheat Bread | Sara Lee
Cereal and Grain Products	1 1/2 cups	Brown Rice, Long Grain, Cooked
Cereals, Ready to Eat	2 tablespoons	Cereal, Rte, Granola, Lowfat-original | Kellogg's
Dairy Products	1/4 cups	Cheddar Cheese, Mild, Shredded, Reduced Fat | Kraft
	1/2 cups	Cheddar Cheese, Double, Shredded | Sargento
	1/2 cups	Yogurt, Greek-style | Cascade Fresh
	3/4 cups	Cheese, Cottage 1%
	1 large	Egg, Chicken, Scrambled
	1 slice	Cheddar Cheese, Medium, Slice | Sargento
	1 1/2 tablespoons	American Cheese | Boar's Head
	3 1/4 cups	Yogurt, Plain, Nonfat | Stonyfield Farm
	3 large	Egg, Chicken, Poached
	3 teaspoons	Butter
	5 1/4 tablespoons	Cheddar Cheese, Sharp, Reduced Fat | Cracker Barrel
Fats and Oils	3 teaspoons	Olive Oil, Extra Virgin | Bertolli
Finfish and Shellfish Products	3/4 oz	Salmon, Sockeye, Baked Or Broiled
	2 oz	Salmon, Atlantic, Wild, Baked Or Broiled
	3 oz	Albacore Tuna In Water, Chunk White, Canned, Lower Sodium | Chicken of the Sea

Continued on next page...

Meal Plan Shopping List

Category	Quantity	Item
Fruits	1/2 oz	Rasin
	1 1/2 cups	Blackberry, Raw
	4 small	Apple W/skin, Raw
	5 small	Banana, Raw
	6 fruit	Nectarine, Raw
	22 large	Strawberry, Raw
Ingredients	2 teaspoons	Balsamic Vinegar	Spectrum
Legumes	1/2 cups	Bean, Navy, Canned
	4 tablespoons	Hummus (seasoned Mashed Chickpea)
	4 1/2 tablespoons	Hummus, Original	Guiltless Gourmet
Nuts and Seeds	5 1/4 tablespoons	Almond Butter, No Salt
Pork	1 oz	Bacon, Canadian-style, Grilled
	4 oz	Pork Center Loin, Braised, Slo
Poultry	3 oz	Chicken, Broiler, Breast, Meat, Roasted
Side Dishes	1 cups	Mixed Vegetables, Frozen	Cascadian Farm
	2 1/2 cups	Quinoa, Cooked
Snacks	3 1/2 oz	Pretzel, Sticks	Rold Gold
	16 1/4 tablespoons	Brown Rice Cake, Corn
Vegetables	1/4 cups	Spinach, Chopped, Frozen	Flav-R-Pac
	3/4 cups	Mustard Greens, Boiled, Drained
	1 1/4 cups	Sweet Potato, Baked, No Salt
	4 cups	Carrot, Baby, Raw
	4 cups	Lettuce, Cos Or Romaine, Raw
	4 leaf	Lettuce, Cos Or Romaine, Raw
	5 oz	Tomato, Raw
	7 oz	Brussels Sprouts, Boiled, No Salt
	12 oz	Squash, Summer, Crookneck, Boiled, Drained

Recipe Shopping List

Category	Quantity	Item
Beverages	2 tablespoons	Lemon Juice
Fats and Oils	4 tablespoons	Olive Oil
Fruits	1 teaspoons	Lemon Peel, Raw
Ingredients	1/4 teaspoons	Salt, Sea
Poultry	6 oz	Chicken Breast, Boneless, Roasted, Meat Only
	16 oz	Chicken, Breast W/o Skin, Raw
Spices	1 tablespoons	Garlic Powder
	1 tablespoons	Sage, Ground
	2 dash	Pepper, Black, Ground
Vegetables	4 cups	Kale, Raw

2250 Calorie Meal Plan

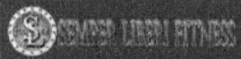
SEMPER LIBERI FITNESS

Meal Plan
SLF Monthly Meal Plan

Prepared By: James Mullins
Email: semperliberifitness@gmail.com
Created: 10-11-2015

SLF Monthly Plan

Day 1

Day 1

Time	Meal Label	Calories	Meal Items
07:00 am	Breakfast	92	2 tablespoons RAISIN
		131	1 1/2 cups OAT BRAN, COOKED
		147	2 large EGG, CHICKEN, POACHED
		0	16 fl oz WATER, DRINKING WATER, PURIFIED
		110	1 cups ORANGE JUICE
Notes:			
Meal Totals: Calories: 480	Carbs: 65g (59%)	Protein: 27g (19%)	Fat: 14g (22%) Fluid: 38oz
10:00 am	Snack	0	16 fl oz WATER, DRINKING WATER, PURIFIED
		112	2 tablespoons CEREAL, RTE, GRANOLA, LOWFAT ORIGINAL
		60	1 fruit NECTARINE, RAW
		127	2/3 cups YOGURT, VANILLA, LOWFAT
Notes:			
Meal Totals: Calories: 299	Carbs: 57g (77%)	Protein: 10g (14%)	Fat: 3g (9%) Fluid: 22oz
12:00 pm	Lunch	33	1 teaspoons MAYONNAISE, OLIVE OIL, ARTISAN
		101	1 oz PRETZEL STICKS
		90	2 oz CHICKEN, BROILER, BREAST, MEAT, ROASTED
		80	1 slice CHEDDAR CHEESE, MEDIUM, SLICE
		2	1 leaf LETTUCE, COS OR ROMAINE, RAW
		160	2 slice 100% WHOLE WHEAT BREAD
		5	1 teaspoons MUSTARD, PREPARED, DIJON
		0	16 fl oz WATER, DRINKING WATER, PURIFIED
		4	1 oz TOMATO, RAW
Notes:			
Meal Totals: Calories: 475	Carbs: 53g (46%)	Protein: 34g (29%)	Fat: 13g (25%) Fluid: 21oz
03:00 pm	Snack	91	1 cups MILK, COW'S, NONFAT VIT-D ADDED (SKIM)
		90	1 small BANANA, RAW
		0	8 fl oz WATER, DRINKING WATER, PURIFIED
		140	1 bar GRANOLA BAR, CHEWY, HONEY ALMOND FLAX
Notes:			
Meal Totals: Calories: 321	Carbs: 55g (65%)	Protein: 16g (19%)	Fat: 6g (16%) Fluid: 19oz
06:00 pm	Dinner	71	3 oz HALIBUT, ATLANTIC & PACIFIC, BAKED OR BROILED
		224	1 cups QUINOA, COOKED
		80	2 teaspoons OLIVE OIL, EXTRA VIRGIN
		41	4 oz BRUSSELS SPROUTS, BOILED, NO SALT
		0	16 fl oz WATER, DRINKING WATER, PURIFIED
Notes:			

SLF Monthly Plan

Day 1

Day 1

Time	Meal Label	Calories	Meal Items
Meal Totals: Calories: 416	Carbs: 47g (44%)	Protein: 25g (24%)	Fat: 15g (32%) Fluid: 22oz
08:00 pm	Snack	172	1 cups CHEESE, COTTAGE 1%
		0	8 fl oz WATER, DRINKING WATER, PURIFIED
		40	1/4 cups WHIPPED CREAM TOPPING, LIGHT
		46	8 large STRAWBERRY, RAW
Notes:			
Meal Totals: Calories: 258	Carbs: 24g (36%)	Protein: 32g (48%)	Fat: 5g (17%) Fluid: 20oz

	Calories	Carbs	Protein	Fat	Fluid
Day 1 Totals:	2249	321g (54%)	144g (24%)	56g (21%)	142oz

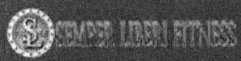
Meal Plan
SLF Monthly Meal Plan

Prepared By: James Mullins
Email: semperliberifitness@gmail.com
Created: 10-11-2015

SLF Monthly Plan

Day 2

Day 2

Time	Meal Label	Calories	Meal Items
07:00 am	Breakfast	147	2 large EGG, CHICKEN, POACHED
		137	1 1/2 cups MILK, COW'S, NONFAT VIT-D ADDED (SKIM)
		0	16 fl oz WATER, DRINKING WATER, PURIFIED
		155	1 1/2 cups WHEAT CHEX, RTE
Notes:			
	Meal Totals:	Calories: 439	Carbs: 53g (47%) Protein: 33g (29%) Fat: 12g (24%) Fluid: 31oz
10:00 am	Snack	101	1 oz PRETZEL STICKS
		152	1 1/2 tablespoons ALMOND BUTTER, NO SALT
		0	16 fl oz WATER, DRINKING WATER, PURIFIED
		55	1 small APPLE W/SKIN, RAW
Notes:			
	Meal Totals:	Calories: 308	Carbs: 43g (53%) Protein: 6g (7%) Fat: 14g (40%) Fluid: 21oz
12:00 pm	Lunch	120	4 oz ALBACORE TUNA IN WATER, CHUNK WHITE, CANNED, LOWER SODIUM
		2	1 leaf LETTUCE, COS OR ROMAINE, RAW
		0	16 fl oz WATER, DRINKING WATER, PURIFIED
		83	1 cups CARROT, BABY, RAW
		67	2 teaspoons MAYONNAISE, OLIVE OIL, ARTISAN
		151	2 pita BREAD, PITA, WHOLE WHEAT
Notes:			
	Meal Totals:	Calories: 423	Carbs: 31g (32%) Protein: 42g (44%) Fat: 10g (24%) Fluid: 21oz
03:00 pm	Snack	140	1 bar GRANOLA BAR, CHEWY, HONEY ALMOND FLAX
		113	1/2 cups YOGURT, ORIGINAL, FRUIT FLAVORS
		60	1 fruit NECTARINE, RAW
		0	16 fl oz WATER, DRINKING WATER, PURIFIED
Notes:			
	Meal Totals:	Calories: 313	Carbs: 57g (72%) Protein: 9g (11%) Fat: 6g (17%) Fluid: 21oz
06:00 pm	Dinner	211	8 oz POTATO, BAKED, FLESH & SKIN
		92	3 oz BEEF, LOIN, T-BONE STEAK, LEAN, 0 TRIM, BROILED
		75	1 roll ROLL, DINNER, WHOLE WHEAT
		22	1 cups MUSTARD GREENS, BOILED, DRAINED
		35	1 teaspoons BUTTER
		0	16 fl oz WATER, DRINKING WATER, PURIFIED
Notes:			
	Meal Totals:	Calories: 435	Carbs: 65g (59%) Protein: 25g (23%) Fat: 9g (18%) Fluid: 31oz

Continued on next page.

SLF Monthly Plan

Day 2

Day 2

Time	Meal Label	Calories	Meal Items
08:00 pm	Snack	90	1 small BANANA, RAW
		0	8 fl oz WATER, DRINKING WATER, PURIFIED
		143	3/4 cups YOGURT, VANILLA, LOWFAT
		112	2 tablespoons CEREAL, RTE, GRANOLA, LOWFAT-ORIGINAL
Notes:			
	Meal Totals:	Calories: 345	Carbs: 68g (77%) Protein: 11g (13%) Fat: 4g (10%) Fluid: 12oz

	Calories	Carbs	Protein	Fat	Fluid
Day 2 Totals:	2263	317g (56%)	126g (22%)	55g (22%)	137oz

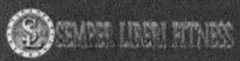
Meal Plan
SLF Monthly Meal Plan

Prepared By: **James Mullins**
Email: **semperliberifitness@gmail.com**
Created: **10-11-2015**

SLF Monthly Plan

Day 3

Day 3

Time	Meal Label	Calories	Meal Items
07:00 am	Breakfast	160	2 slice 100% WHOLE WHEAT BREAD
		0	16 fl oz WATER, DRINKING WATER, PURIFIED
		60	1 fruit NECTARINE, RAW
		91	1 cups MILK, COW'S, NONFAT VIT-D ADDED (SKIM)
		203	2 tablespoons ALMOND BUTTER, NO SALT
Notes:			
	Meal Totals	**Calories: 514**	**Carbs: 60g (45%) Protein: 24g (18%) Fat: 22g (37%) Fluid: 30oz**
10:00 am	Snack	86	1/2 cups CHEESE, COTTAGE 1%
		0	16 fl oz WATER, DRINKING WATER, PURIFIED
		140	1 bar GRANOLA BAR, CHEWY, HONEY ALMOND FLAX
		55	1 small APPLE W/SKIN, RAW
Notes:			
	Meal Totals	**Calories: 281**	**Carbs: 39g (54%) Protein: 20g (28%) Fat: 6g (19%) Fluid: 24oz**
12:00 pm	Lunch	75	1 roll ROLL, DINNER, WHOLE WHEAT
		2	1 teaspoons BALSAMIC VINEGAR
		40	1 teaspoons OLIVE OIL, EXTRA VIRGIN
		16	2 cups LETTUCE, COS OR ROMAINE, RAW
		8	2 oz TOMATO, RAW
		92	3 oz BEEF, LOIN, T-BONE STEAK, LEAN, 0 TRIM, BROILED
		2	16 fl oz ICED TEA, UNSWEETENED
		168	3/4 cups QUINOA, COOKED
Notes:			
	Meal Totals	**Calories: 403**	**Carbs: 48g (48%) Protein: 23g (23%) Fat: 13g (29%) Fluid: 26oz**
03:00 pm	Snack	83	1 cups CARROT, BABY, RAW
		108	4 tablespoons HUMMUS (SEASONED MASHED CHICKPEA)
		0	16 fl oz WATER, DRINKING WATER, PURIFIED
		101	1 oz PRETZEL, STICKS
Notes:			
	Meal Totals	**Calories: 292**	**Carbs: 35g (68%) Protein: 5g (10%) Fat: 5g (22%) Fluid: 18oz**
06:00 pm	Dinner	218	SAGE & GARLIC ROASTED CHICKEN (TOTALS) (1 Servings)
		162	3/4 cups BROWN RICE, LONG GRAIN, COOKED
		18	4 oz SQUASH, SUMMER, CROOKNECK, BOILED, DRAINED
		0	16 fl oz WATER, DRINKING WATER, PURIFIED
		75	1 pita BREAD, PITA, WHOLE WHEAT
Notes:			

Continued on next page...

SLF Monthly Plan

Day 3

Day 3

Time	Meal Label	Calories	Meal Items		
	Meal Totals	**Calories: 473**	**Carbs: 56g (47%) Protein: 35g (29%) Fat: 13g (24%) Fluid: 24oz**		
08:00 pm	Snack	190	1 cups YOGURT, VANILLA, LOWFAT		
		31	1/2 cups BLACKBERRY, RAW		
		56	1 tablespoons CEREAL, RTE, GRANOLA, LOWFAT-ORIGINAL		
		0	8 fl oz WATER, DRINKING WATER, PURIFIED		
Notes:					
	Meal Totals	**Calories: 277**	**Carbs: 49g (71%) Protein: 13g (19%) Fat: 3g (10%) Fluid: 12oz**		
		Calories	Carbs	Protein	Fat	Fluid
	Day 3 Totals:	**2240**	**287g (53%)**	**120g (22%)**	**62g (26%)**	**134oz**

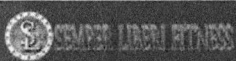
Meal Plan
SLF Monthly Meal Plan

Prepared By: **James Mullins**
Email: **semperliberifitness@gmail.com**
Created: **10-11-2015**

SLF Monthly Plan   **Day 4**

Day 4

Time	Meal Label	Calories	Meal Items
07:00 am	Breakfast	110	1 cups ORANGE JUICE
		0	16 fl oz WATER, DRINKING WATER, PURIFIED
		170	1 wrap WRAP, 100% WHOLE WHEAT
		10	2 tablespoons SALSA
		203	2 large EGG, CHICKEN, SCRAMBLED
Notes:			
	Meal Totals:	Calories: 493	Carbs: 57g (46%) Protein: 21g (17%) Fat: 21g (38%) Fluid: 29oz
10:00 am	Snack	129	3/4 cups CHEESE, COTTAGE 1%
		0	16 fl oz WATER, DRINKING WATER, PURIFIED
		60	1 fruit NECTARINE, RAW
		51	1/2 oz PRETZEL, STICKS
Notes:			
	Meal Totals:	Calories: 240	Carbs: 31g (51%) Protein: 25g (41%) Fat: 2g (7%) Fluid: 27oz
12:00 pm	Lunch	218	SAGE & GARLIC ROASTED CHICKEN (TOTALS) (1 Servings)
		168	3/4 cups QUINOA, COOKED
		90	1 cups MIXED VEGETABLES, FROZEN
		0	16 fl oz WATER, DRINKING WATER, PURIFIED
		75	1 roll ROLL, DINNER, WHOLE WHEAT
		17	1/2 teaspoons BUTTER
Notes:			
	Meal Totals:	Calories: 568	Carbs: 63g (45%) Protein: 38g (27%) Fat: 17g (27%) Fluid: 18oz
03:00 pm	Snack	92	1 oz RAISIN
		46	1/2 cups MILK, COW'S, NONFAT VIT D ADDED (SKIM)
		140	1 bar GRANOLA BAR, CHEWY, HONEY ALMOND FLAX
		0	12 fl oz WATER, DRINKING WATER, PURIFIED
Notes:			
	Meal Totals:	Calories: 278	Carbs: 47g (68%) Protein: 11g (16%) Fat: 5g (16%) Fluid: 17oz
06:00 pm	Dinner	162	3/4 cups BROWN RICE, LONG GRAIN, COOKED
		156	1/2 cups BEAN, NAVY, CANNED
		0	16 fl oz WATER, DRINKING WATER, PURIFIED
		17	3/4 cups MUSTARD GREENS, BOILED, DRAINED
		115	2 oz PORK CENTER LOIN, BRAISED, SLO
Notes:			
	Meal Totals:	Calories: 450	Carbs: 64g (56%) Protein: 34g (30%) Fat: 7g (14%) Fluid: 30oz

Continued on next page...

SLF Monthly Plan   **Day 4**

Day 4

Time	Meal Label	Calories	Meal Items			
08:00 pm	Snack	143	3/4 cups YOGURT, VANILLA, LOWFAT			
		90	1 small BANANA, RAW			
		0	8 fl oz WATER, DRINKING WATER, PURIFIED			
Notes:						
	Meal Totals:	Calories: 233	Carbs: 46g (77%) Protein: 9g (15%) Fat: 2g (8%) Fluid: 11oz			
		Calories	Carbs	Protein	Fat	Fluid
	Day 4 Totals:	2262	308g (54%)	138g (24%)	54g (21%)	132oz

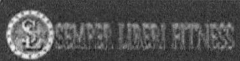
Meal Plan
SLF Monthly Meal Plan

Prepared By: James Mullins
Email: semperliberifitness@gmail.com
Created: 10-11-2015

SLF Monthly Plan Day 5

Day 5

Time	Meal Label	Calories	Meal Items
07:00 am	Breakfast	159	1 1/2 cups WHEAT CHEX, RTE
		0	16 fl oz WATER, DRINKING WATER, PURIFIED
		52	1 oz BACON, CANADIAN-STYLE, GRILLED
		101	1 large EGG, CHICKEN, SCRAMBLED
		183	2 cups MILK, COWS, NONFAT VIT-D ADDED (SKIM)
Notes:			
Meal Totals:	**Calories: 493**	**Carbs: 58g (48%) Protein: 39g (32%) Fat: 11g (20%) Fluid: 35oz**	
10:00 am	Snack	55	1 small APPLE W/SKIN, RAW
		0	16 fl oz WATER, DRINKING WATER, PURIFIED
		203	2 tablespoons ALMOND BUTTER, NO SALT
Notes:			
Meal Totals:	**Calories: 258**	**Carbs: 22g (32%) Protein: 5g (7%) Fat: 19g (61%) Fluid: 21oz**	
12:00 pm	Lunch	0	16 fl oz WATER, DRINKING WATER, PURIFIED
		2	1 teaspoons BALSAMIC VINEGAR
		75	1 rol ROLL, DINNER, WHOLE WHEAT
		211	8 oz POTATO, BAKED, FLESH & SKIN
		16	2 cups LETTUCE, COS OR ROMAINE, RAW
		40	1 teaspoons OLIVE OIL, EXTRA VIRGIN
		143	2 1/2 oz PORK CENTER LOIN, BRAISED, SLO
Notes:			
Meal Totals:	**Calories: 487**	**Carbs: 66g (54%) Protein: 30g (24%) Fat: 12g (22%) Fluid: 29oz**	
03:00 pm	Snack	0	16 fl oz WATER, DRINKING WATER, PURIFIED
		83	1 cups CARROT, BABY, RAW
		101	1 oz PRETZEL, STICKS
		54	2 tablespoons HUMMUS (SEASONED MASHED CHICKPEA)
Notes:			
Meal Totals:	**Calories: 238**	**Carbs: 29g (75%) Protein: 3g (8%) Fat: 3g (17%) Fluid: 17oz**	
06:00 pm	Dinner	320	CHOPPED KALE SALAD WITH CHICKEN (TOTALS) (1 Servings)
		151	2 pita BREAD, PITA, WHOLE WHEAT
		0	16 fl oz WATER, DRINKING WATER, PURIFIED
Notes:			
Meal Totals:	**Calories: 471**	**Carbs: 46g (38%) Protein: 46g (38%) Fat: 13g (24%) Fluid: 17oz**	

Continued on next page...

SLF Monthly Plan Day 5

Day 5

Time	Meal Label	Calories	Meal Items
08:00 pm	Snack	140	1 bar GRANOLA BAR, CHEWY, HONEY ALMOND FLAX
		0	8 fl oz WATER, DRINKING WATER, PURIFIED
		90	1 small BANANA, RAW
		95	1/2 cups YOGURT, VANILLA, LOWFAT
Notes:			
Meal Totals:	**Calories: 325**	**Carbs: 60g (70%) Protein: 12g (14%) Fat: 6g (16%) Fluid: 11oz**	

		Calories	Carbs	Protein	Fat	Fluid
	Day 5 Totals:	2270	281g (50%)	135g (24%)	64g (26%)	130oz

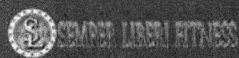
Meal Plan
SLF Monthly Meal Plan

Prepared By: James Mullins
Email: semperliberifitness@gmail.com
Created: 10-11-2015

SLF Monthly Plan   Day 6

Day 6

Time	Meal Label	Calories	Meal Items
07:00 am	Breakfast	160	2 slice 100% WHOLE WHEAT BREAD
		101	1 tablespoons ALMOND BUTTER, NO SALT
		90	1 small BANANA, RAW
		0	16 fl oz WATER, DRINKING WATER, PURIFIED
		137	1 1/2 cups MILK, COW'S, NONFAT VIT-D ADDED (SKIM)
Notes:			
	Meal Totals:	**Calories: 488**	Carbs: 70g (57%) Protein: 26g (21%) Fat: 12g (22%) Fluid: 31oz
10:00 am	Snack	0	16 fl oz WATER, DRINKING WATER, PURIFIED
		238	1 1/4 cups YOGURT, VANILLA, LOWFAT
		60	1 fruit NECTARINE, RAW
Notes:			
	Meal Totals:	**Calories: 298**	Carbs: 53g (71%) Protein: 15g (20%) Fat: 3g (9%) Fluid: 23oz
12:00 pm	Lunch	320	CHOPPED KALE SALAD WITH CHICKEN (TOTALS) (1 Servings)
		2	16 fl oz ICED TEA, UNSWEETENED
		75	1 roll ROLL, DINNER, WHOLE WHEAT
		35	1 teaspoons BUTTER
Notes:			
	Meal Totals:	**Calories: 432**	Carbs: 28g (27%) Protein: 42g (38%) Fat: 17g (35%) Fluid: 19oz
03:00 pm	Snack	140	1 bar GRANOLA BAR, CHEWY, HONEY ALMOND FLAX
		55	1 small APPLE W/SKIN, RAW
		0	16 fl oz WATER, DRINKING WATER, PURIFIED
		101	1 oz PRETZEL, STICKS
Notes:			
	Meal Totals:	**Calories: 296**	Carbs: 59g (76%) Protein: 7g (9%) Fat: 5g (15%) Fluid: 20oz
06:00 pm	Dinner	154	5 oz SALMON, ATLANTIC, WILD, BAKED OR BROILED
		216	1 cups BROWN RICE, LONG GRAIN, COOKED
		0	16 fl oz WATER, DRINKING WATER, PURIFIED
		69	2 teaspoons BUTTER
		27	6 oz SQUASH, SUMMER, CROOKNECK, BOILED, DRAINED
Notes:			
	Meal Totals:	**Calories: 466**	Carbs: 51g (43%) Protein: 28g (24%) Fat: 17g (33%) Fluid: 30oz
08:00 pm	Snack	112	2 tablespoons CEREAL, RTE, GRANOLA, LOWFAT-ORIGINAL
		46	8 large STRAWBERRY, RAW
		0	8 fl oz WATER, DRINKING WATER, PURIFIED
		129	3/4 cups CHEESE, COTTAGE 1%

Continued on next page...

SLF Monthly Plan   Day 6

Day 6

Time	Meal Label	Calories	Meal Items
Notes:			
	Meal Totals:	**Calories: 287**	Carbs: 38g (52%) Protein: 26g (36%) Fat: 4g (12%) Fluid: 20oz

	Calories	Carbs	Protein	Fat	Fluid
Day 6 Totals:	2267	300g (52%)	144g (25%)	58g (23%)	141oz

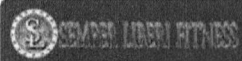

Meal Plan
SLF Monthly Meal Plan

Prepared By: **James Mullins**
Email: **semperliberifitness@gmail.com**
Created: **10-11-2015**

SLF Monthly Plan Day 7

Day 7

Time	Meal Label	Calories	Meal Items
07:00 am	Breakfast	169	1 1/4 muffin ENGLISH MUFFIN, WHOLE WHEAT, TOASTED
		0	16 fl oz WATER, DRINKING WATER, PURIFIED
		35	1 teaspoons BUTTER
		110	1 cups ORANGE JUICE
		147	2 large EGG, CHICKEN, POACHED
Notes:			
	Meal Totals:	Calories: 461	Carbs: 60g (50%) Protein: 22g (18%) Fat: 17g (32%) Fluid: 30oz
10:00 am	Snack	0	16 fl oz WATER, DRINKING WATER, PURIFIED
		83	1 cups CARROT, BABY, RAW
		70	1/2 cups BLACK BEAN
		101	1 oz PRETZEL, STICKS
Notes:			
	Meal Totals:	Calories: 254	Carbs: 40g (65%) Protein: 7g (15%) Fat: 0g (0%) Fluid: 16oz
12:00 pm	Lunch	340	2 wrap WRAP, 100% WHOLE WHEAT
		33	1 teaspoons MAYONNAISE, OLIVE OIL, ARTISAN
		3	2 leaf LETTUCE, COS OR ROMAINE, RAW
		10	2 teaspoons MUSTARD, PREPARED, DIJON
		8	2 oz TOMATO, RAW
		0	16 fl oz WATER, DRINKING WATER, PURIFIED
		161	3 oz TURKEY BREAST, ROASTED
Notes:			
	Meal Totals:	Calories: 555	Carbs: 58g (43%) Protein: 34g (25%) Fat: 19g (32%) Fluid: 22oz
03:00 pm	Snack	35	6 large STRAWBERRY, RAW
		0	16 fl oz WATER, DRINKING WATER, PURIFIED
		143	3/4 cups YOGURT, VANILLA, LOWFAT
		112	2 tablespoons CEREAL, RTE, GRANOLA, LOWFAT-ORIGINAL
Notes:			
	Meal Totals:	Calories: 290	Carbs: 53g (73%) Protein: 11g (15%) Fat: 4g (12%) Fluid: 21oz
06:00 pm	Dinner	41	4 oz BRUSSELS SPROUTS, BOILED, NO SALT
		0	16 fl oz WATER, DRINKING WATER, PURIFIED
		224	1 cups QUINOA, COOKED
		35	1 teaspoons BUTTER
		160	4 oz CHICKEN, BROILER, BREAST, MEAT, ROASTED
Notes:			
	Meal Totals:	Calories: 460	Carbs: 47g (39%) Protein: 46g (40%) Fat: 11g (21%) Fluid: 24oz

Continued on next page...

SLF Monthly Plan Day 7

Day 7

Time	Meal Label	Calories	Meal Items
08:00 pm	Snack	0	8 fl oz WATER, DRINKING WATER, PURIFIED
		90	1 small BANANA, RAW
		140	1 bar GRANOLA BAR, CHEWY, HONEY ALMOND FLAX
Notes:			
	Meal Totals:	Calories: 230	Carbs: 44g (72%) Protein: 6g (10%) Fat: 5g (18%) Fluid: 11oz

		Calories	Carbs	Protein	Fat	Fluid
	Day 7 Totals:	2270	302g (54%)	128g (23%)	56g (23%)	124oz

Sage & Garlic Roasted Chicken (totals) (serves 4)

Ingredients

- 1 tablespoons Garlic Powder
- 1 tablespoons Sage, Ground
- 3 tablespoons Olive Oil
- 2 dash Pepper, Black, Ground
- 16 oz Chicken, Breast W/o Skin, Raw

Instructions

Preheat oven to 375. Wash chicken inside and out, pat dry with paper towels. In a small bowl, whisk together sage, oil, garlic and pepper. Rub this mixture under the skin of the breast and on the skin all over the chicken. Place chicken, breast side down, on lightly greased pan. Roast for 30 minutes, then turn chicken breast side up and continue roasting until internal temperature reaches 180.

Chopped Kale Salad with Chicken (totals) (serves 2)

Ingredients

- 4 cups Kale, Raw
- 1 teaspoons Lemon Peel, Raw
- 8 oz Chicken Breast, Boneless, Roasted, Meat Only
- 1 tablespoons Olive Oil
- 1/4 teaspoons Salt, Sea
- 2 tablespoons Lemon Juice

Instructions

1. Combine olive oil, lemon juice, lemon zest, salt, and pepper in small bowl.

2. Pour over chopped kale and toss.

3. Divide kale into 2 bowls.

4. Top each bowl of kale with 4 oz of roasted chicken breast.

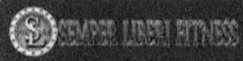

Meal Plan Shopping List

Category	Quantity	Item
Accompaniments	1/4 cups	Whipped Cream Topping, Light | Cool Whip
	2 tablespoons	Salsa
	3 teaspoons	Mustard, Prepared, Dijon | Grey Poupon
	4 teaspoons	Mayonnaise, Olive Oil, Artisan | Spectrum
Beef	6 oz	Beef, Loin, T-bone Steak, Lean, 0 Trim, Broiled
Beverages	3 cups	Orange Juice
	7 1/2 cups	Milk, Cow's, Nonfat Vit-d Added (skim)
	32 fl oz	Iced Tea, Unsweetened | Generic
	572 fl oz	Water, Drinking Water, Purified
Bread	1 1/4 muffin	English Muffin, Whole Wheat, Toasted
	3 wrap	Wrap, 100% Whole Wheat | Sahara
	5 pita	Bread, Pita, Whole Wheat
	5 roll	Roll, Dinner, Whole Wheat
	6 slice	100% Whole Wheat Bread | Sara Lee
Cereal and Grain Products	1 1/2 cups	Oat Bran, Cooked
	2 1/2 cups	Brown Rice, Long Grain, Cooked
Cereals, Ready to Eat	3 cups	Wheat Chex, Rte | Ralston
	9 tablespoons	Cereal, Rte, Granola, Lowfat-original | Kellogg's
Dairy Products	1/2 cups	Yogurt, Original, Fruit Flavors | Yoplait
	1 slice	Cheddar Cheese, Medium, Slice | Sargento
	3 cups	Cheese, Cottage 1%
	5 2/3 cups	Yogurt, Vanilla, Lowfat | Mountain High
	3 large	Egg, Chicken, Scrambled
	6 large	Egg, Chicken, Poached
	6 1/2 teaspoons	Butter
Fats and Oils	4 teaspoons	Olive Oil, Extra Virgin | Bertolli
Finfish and Shellfish Products	3 oz	Halibut, Atlantic & Pacific, Baked Or Broiled
	4 oz	Albacore Tuna in Water, Chunk White, Canned, Lower Sodium | Chicken of the Sea
	5 oz	Salmon, Atlantic, Wild, Baked Or Broiled
Fruits	1/2 cups	Blackberry, Raw
	2 oz	Raisin
	4 small	Apple W/skin, Raw
	5 fruit	Nectarine, Raw
	6 small	Banana, Raw
	22 large	Strawberry, Raw

Continued on next page

Meal Plan Shopping List

Category	Quantity	Item
Ingredients	2 teaspoons	Balsamic Vinegar	Spectrum
Legumes	1/2 cups	Bean, Navy, Canned
	1/2 cups	Black Bean	S&W
	6 tablespoons	Hummus (seasoned Mashed Chickpea)
Nuts and Seeds	6 1/2 tablespoons	Almond Butter, No Salt
Pork	1 oz	Bacon, Canadian-style, Grilled
	4 1/2 oz	Pork Center Loin, Braised, Slo
Poultry	3 oz	Turkey Breast, Roasted
	6 oz	Chicken, Broiler, Breast, Meat, Roasted
Side Dishes	1 cups	Mixed Vegetables, Frozen	Cascadian Farm
	3 1/2 cups	Quinoa, Cooked
Snacks	6 1/2 oz	Pretzel, Sticks	Rold Gold
	7 bar	Granola Bar, Chewy, Honey Almond Flax	Kashi
Vegetables	1 3/4 cups	Mustard Greens, Boiled, Drained
	4 cups	Carrot, Baby, Raw
	4 cups	Lettuce, Cos Or Romaine, Raw
	4 leaf	Lettuce, Cos Or Romaine, Raw
	5 oz	Tomato, Raw
	8 oz	Brussels Sprouts, Boiled, No Salt
	8 oz	Potato, Baked, Flesh & Skin
	8 oz	Potato, Baked, Flesh & Skin
	10 oz	Squash, Summer, Crookneck, Boiled, Drained

Recipe Shopping List

Category	Quantity	Item
Beverages	2 tablespoons	Lemon Juice
Fats and Oils	4 tablespoons	Olive Oil
Fruits	1 teaspoons	Lemon Peel, Raw
Ingredients	1/4 teaspoons	Salt, Sea
Poultry	8 oz	Chicken Breast, Boneless, Roasted, Meat Only
	16 oz	Chicken, Breast W/o Skin, Raw
Spices	1 tablespoons	Garlic Powder
	1 tablespoons	Sage, Ground
	2 dash	Pepper, Black, Ground
Vegetables	4 cups	Kale, Raw

3000 Calorie Meal Plan

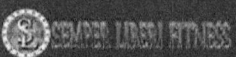 SEMPER LIBERI FITNESS   *Become Free*

Meal Plan
SLF Monthly Meal Plan

Prepared By: **James Mullins**
Email: semperliberifitness@gmail.com
Created: 10-11-2015

SLF Monthly Plan   Day 1

Day 1

Time	Meal Label	Calories	Meal Items
07:00 am	Breakfast	35	1 teaspoons BUTTER
		120	1 muffin ENGLISH MUFFIN, 100% WHOLE WHEAT
		83	1 cups BLUEBERRY, RAW
		155	2 egg EGG, CHICKEN, WHOLE, HARD, BOILED
		0	16 fl oz WATER, DRINKING WATER, PURIFIED
		300	1 cups OATS, ROLLED, OLD FASHIONED (OATMEAL)

Notes:

| Meal Totals: | Calories: 693 | Carbs: 99g (55%) | Protein: 30g (17%) | Fat: 22g (28%) | Fluid: 25oz |

Time	Meal Label	Calories	Meal Items
10:00 am	Snack	203	2 tablespoons ALMOND BUTTER, NO SALT
		55	1 small APPLE W/SKIN, RAW
		82	3/4 cups MILK, FLUID, PART SKIM, 1% BF

Notes:

| Meal Totals: | Calories: 340 | Carbs: 31g (34%) | Protein: 12g (13%) | Fat: 21g (52%) | Fluid: 11oz |

Time	Meal Label	Calories	Meal Items
12:00 pm	Lunch	176	20 crackers CRACKER, WHEAT THIN, BAKED
		268	5 oz TURKEY BREAST, ROASTED
		151	2 pita BREAD, PITA, WHOLE WHEAT
		83	1 cups CARROT, BABY, RAW
		2	1 leaf LETTUCE, COS OR ROMAINE, RAW
		8	2 oz TOMATO, RAW
		0	16 fl oz WATER, DRINKING WATER, PURIFIED

Notes:

| Meal Totals: | Calories: 688 | Carbs: 58g (38%) | Protein: 50g (33%) | Fat: 20g (29%) | Fluid: 25oz |

Time	Meal Label	Calories	Meal Items
03:00 pm	Snack	187	10 toasts CRACKER, MELBA TOAST, WHEAT
		90	1 small BANANA, RAW
		0	16 fl oz WATER, DRINKING WATER, PURIFIED
		80	1 piece STRING CHEESE

Notes:

| Meal Totals: | Calories: 357 | Carbs: 62g (68%) | Protein: 14g (15%) | Fat: 7g (17%) | Fluid: 20oz |

Time	Meal Label	Calories	Meal Items
06:00 pm	Dinner	226	3/4 cups BEAN, BLACK, BOILED
		147	4 oz TILAPIA, FRESH
		0	16 fl oz WATER, DRINKING WATER, PURIFIED
		83	1 cups BROCCOLI, BOILED, NO SALT
		162	3/4 cups BROWN RICE, LONG GRAIN, COOKED

Notes:

| Meal Totals: | Calories: 618 | Carbs: 92g (58%) | Protein: 53g (33%) | Fat: 6g (9%) | Fluid: 32oz |

Continued on next page...

SLF Monthly Plan   Day 1

Day 1

Time	Meal Label	Calories	Meal Items
08:00 pm	Snack	90	1 bars GRANOLA BAR, OATS 'N HONEY
		61	1 large PEACH, RAW
		0	8 fl oz WATER, DRINKING WATER, PURIFIED
		179	6 oz YOGURT, FRUIT, LOW FAT

Notes:

| Meal Totals: | Calories: 330 | Carbs: 62g (74%) | Protein: 11g (13%) | Fat: 5g (13%) | Fluid: 19oz |

	Calories	Carbs	Protein	Fat	Fluid
Day 1 Totals:	3026	404g (53%)	170g (22%)	81g (24%)	132oz

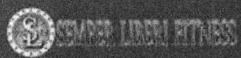
Meal Plan
SLF Monthly Meal Plan

Prepared By: James Mullins
Email: semperliberifitness@gmail.com
Created: 10-11-2015

SLF Monthly Plan Day 2

Day 2

Time	Meal Label	Calories	Meal Items
07:00 am	Breakfast	293	2 cups OAT BRAN FLAKES CEREAL, RTE
		155	2 large EGG, CHICKEN, HARD-BOILED
		0	16 fl oz WATER, DRINKING WATER, PURIFIED
		219	16 fl oz MILK, FLUID, PART SKIM, 1% BF
Notes:			
	Meal Totals:	Calories: 667	Carbs: 87g (52%) Protein: 39g (23%) Fat: 19g (25%) Fluid: 34oz
10:00 am	Snack	180	2 bars GRANOLA BAR, OATS 'N HONEY
		129	6 oz GRAPE, RAW
		123	3/4 oz ALMOND, RAW
		0	16 fl oz WATER, DRINKING WATER, PURIFIED
Notes:			
	Meal Totals:	Calories: 432	Carbs: 61g (55%) Protein: 10g (9%) Fat: 18g (36%) Fluid: 23oz
12:00 pm	Lunch	93	4 tablespoons CRANBERRY, DRIED, SWEETENED
		225	5 oz CHICKEN, BROILER, BREAST, MEAT, ROASTED
		0	16 fl oz WATER, DRINKING WATER, PURIFIED
		16	2 cups LETTUCE, COS OR ROMAINE, RAW
		80	2 teaspoons OLIVE OIL, EXTRA VIRGIN
		151	1 roll ROLL, DINNER, WHOLE WHEAT
		4	2 teaspoons BALSAMIC VINEGAR
Notes:			
	Meal Totals:	Calories: 569	Carbs: 58g (40%) Protein: 52g (36%) Fat: 15g (23%) Fluid: 16oz
03:00 pm	Snack	81	1 pear PEAR, RAW
		0	16 fl oz WATER, DRINKING WATER, PURIFIED
		80	1 piece STRING CHEESE
		187	10 toasts CRACKER, MELBA TOAST, WHEAT
Notes:			
	Meal Totals:	Calories: 348	Carbs: 60g (67%) Protein: 14g (16%) Fat: 7g (18%) Fluid: 22oz
06:00 pm	Dinner	151	2 pita BREAD, PITA, WHOLE WHEAT
		0	16 fl oz WATER, DRINKING WATER, PURIFIED
		158	4 oz BEEF, FLANK, FLANK STEAK, LEAN, 0" TRIM, BROILED
		204	8 oz SWEET POTATO, BAKED, NO SALT
		41	1 cups SPINACH, BOILED, NO SALT
Notes:			
	Meal Totals:	Calories: 554	Carbs: 85g (60%) Protein: 38g (27%) Fat: 8g (13%) Fluid: 32oz

Continued on next page.

SLF Monthly Plan Day 2

Day 2

Time	Meal Label	Calories	Meal Items
08:00 pm	Snack	0	8 fl oz WATER, DRINKING WATER, PURIFIED
		164	1 oz ALMOND, RAW
		83	1 cups BLUEBERRY, RAW
		203	1 cups COTTAGE CHEESE, 2% FAT
Notes:			
	Meal Totals:	Calories: 450	Carbs: 35g (31%) Protein: 38g (33%) Fat: 18g (36%) Fluid: 21oz

		Calories	Carbs	Protein	Fat	Fluid
	Day 2 Totals:	3020	386g (50%)	191g (25%)	85g (25%)	158oz

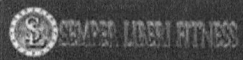

Meal Plan
SLF Monthly Meal Plan

Prepared By: **James Mullins**
Email: **semperliberifitness@gmail.com**
Created: **10-11-2015**

SLF Monthly Plan   **Day 3**

Day 3

Time	Meal Label	Calories	Meal Items
07:00 am	Breakfast	0	16 fl oz WATER, DRINKING WATER, PURIFIED
		240	2 muffin ENGLISH MUFFIN, 100% WHOLE WHEAT
		203	2 tablespoons ALMOND BUTTER, NO SALT
		81	1 pear PEAR, RAW
		110	1 cups MILK, FLUID, PART SKIM, 1% BF
Notes:			
	Meal Totals: Calories: 634	Carbs: 87g (52%)	Protein: 27g (16%) Fat: 24g (32%) Fluid: 30oz
10:00 am	Snack	180	2 bars GRANOLA BAR, OATS 'N HONEY
		0	16 fl oz WATER, DRINKING WATER, PURIFIED
		90	1 small BANANA, RAW
		78	1 egg EGG, CHICKEN, WHOLE, HARD, BOILED
Notes:			
	Meal Totals: Calories: 348	Carbs: 53g (60%)	Protein: 11g (12%) Fat: 11g (28%) Fluid: 22oz
12:00 pm	Lunch	176	20 crackers CRACKER, WHEAT THIN, BAKED
		320	4 slice 100% WHOLE WHEAT BREAD
		55	1 small APPLE W/SKIN, RAW
		0	16 fl oz WATER, DRINKING WATER, PURIFIED
		67	2 teaspoons MAYONNAISE, OLIVE OIL, ARTISAN
		12	3 oz TOMATO, RAW
		3	2 leaf LETTUCE, COS OR ROMAINE, RAW
		120	4 oz ALBACORE TUNA IN WATER, CHUNK WHITE, CANNED, LOWER SODIUM
Notes:			
	Meal Totals: Calories: 753	Carbs: 100g (49%)	Protein: 56g (28%) Fat: 21g (23%) Fluid: 28oz
03:00 pm	Snack	80	1 piece STRING CHEESE
		187	10 toasts CRACKER, MELBA TOAST, WHEAT
		83	1 cups CARROT, BABY, RAW
		0	16 fl oz WATER, DRINKING WATER, PURIFIED
Notes:			
	Meal Totals: Calories: 350	Carbs: 39g (58%)	Protein: 13g (19%) Fat: 7g (23%) Fluid: 17oz
06:00 pm	Dinner	40	1 teaspoons OLIVE OIL, EXTRA VIRGIN
		0	16 fl oz WATER, DRINKING WATER, PURIFIED
		280	**ITALIAN CHICKEN (TOTALS) (1.5 Servings)**
		39	1 cups KALE, BOILED, NO SALT
		248	7 oz PASTA, MACARONI WHOLE WHEAT, COOKED
Notes:			

Continued on next page...

SLF Monthly Plan   **Day 3**

Day 3

Time	Meal Label	Calories	Meal Items		
	Meal Totals: Calories: 607	Carbs: 62g (39%)	Protein: 55g (34%) Fat: 19g (27%) Fluid: 26oz		
08:00 pm	Snack	238	8 oz YOGURT, FRUIT, LOW FAT		
		0	8 fl oz WATER, DRINKING WATER, PURIFIED		
		61	1 large PEACH, RAW		
Notes:					
	Meal Totals: Calories: 299	Carbs: 57g (75%)	Protein: 12g (16%) Fat: 3g (9%) Fluid: 19oz		
		Calories	Carbs	Protein	Fat	Fluid
	Day 3 Totals:	2991	398g (52%)	174g (23%)	85g (25%)	142oz

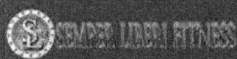
Meal Plan
SLF Monthly Meal Plan

Prepared By: James Mullins
Email: semperliberifitness@gmail.com
Created: 10-11-2015

SLF Monthly Plan   **Day 4**

Day 4

Time	Meal Label	Calories	Meal Items
07:00 am	Breakfast	35	1 teaspoons BUTTER
		0	16 fl oz WATER, DRINKING WATER, PURIFIED
		120	1 muffin ENGLISH MUFFIN, 100% WHOLE WHEAT
		83	1 cups BLUEBERRY, RAW
		155	2 egg EGG, CHICKEN, WHOLE, HARD, BOILED
		300	1 cups OATS, ROLLED, OLD FASHIONED (OATMEAL)

Notes:

| Meal Totals: | Calories: 693 | Carbs: 99g (55%) | Protein: 30g (17%) | Fat: 22g (28%) | Fluid: 25oz |

10:00 am	Snack	164	1 oz ALMOND, RAW
		0	16 fl oz WATER, DRINKING WATER, PURIFIED
		81	1 pear PEAR, RAW
		150	8 toasts CRACKER, MELBA TOAST, WHEAT

Notes:

| Meal Totals: | Calories: 395 | Carbs: 58g (56%) | Protein: 12g (12%) | Fat: 15g (33%) | Fluid: 23oz |

12:00 pm	Lunch	280	ITALIAN CHICKEN (TOTALS) (1.5 Servings)
		8	2 oz TOMATO, RAW
		60	1 1/2 teaspoons OLIVE OIL, EXTRA VIRGIN
		8	1 cups LETTUCE, COS OR ROMAINE, RAW
		283	8 oz PASTA, MACARONI WHOLE WHEAT, COOKED
		2	16 fl oz ICED TEA, UNSWEETENED
		2	1 teaspoons BALSAMIC VINEGAR

Notes:

| Meal Totals: | Calories: 643 | Carbs: 67g (41%) | Protein: 53g (32%) | Fat: 20g (27%) | Fluid: 27oz |

03:00 pm	Snack	180	2 bars GRANOLA BAR, OATS 'N HONEY
		0	16 fl oz WATER, DRINKING WATER, PURIFIED
		145	1 3/4 cups CARROT, BABY, RAW

Notes:

| Meal Totals: | Calories: 325 | Carbs: 29g (62%) | Protein: 4g (9%) | Fat: 6g (29%) | Fluid: 17oz |

06:00 pm	Dinner	151	2 pita BREAD, PITA, WHOLE WHEAT
		29	1 cups ZUCCHINI W/SKIN, BOILED, NO SALT
		0	16 fl oz WATER, DRINKING WATER, PURIFIED
		158	4 oz BEEF, FLANK, FLANK STEAK, LEAN, 0" TRIM, BROILED
		271	1 1/4 cups BROWN RICE, LONG GRAIN, COOKED

Notes:

| Meal Totals: | Calories: 609 | Carbs: 94g (62%) | Protein: 35g (23%) | Fat: 10g (15%) | Fluid: 33oz |

Continued on next page...

SLF Monthly Plan   **Day 4**

Day 4

Time	Meal Label	Calories	Meal Items
08:00 pm	Snack	0	8 fl oz WATER, DRINKING WATER, PURIFIED
		203	1 cups COTTAGE CHEESE, 2% FAT
		129	6 oz GRAPE, RAW

Notes:

| Meal Totals: | Calories: 332 | Carbs: 26g (45%) | Protein: 32g (40%) | Fat: 5g (14%) | Fluid: 2.0oz |

	Calories	Carbs	Protein	Fat	Fluid
Day 4 Totals:	2997	383g (53%)	166g (23%)	78g (24%)	145oz

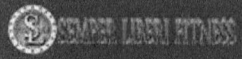
Meal Plan
SLF Monthly Meal Plan

Prepared By: James Mullins
Email: semperliberifitness@gmail.com
Created: 10-11-2015

SLF Monthly Plan

Day 5

Day 5

Time	Meal Label	Calories	Meal Items
07:00 am	Breakfast	155	2 large EGG, CHICKEN, HARD-BOILED
		0	16 fl oz WATER, DRINKING WATER, PURIFIED
		219	16 fl oz MILK, FLUID, PART SKIM, 1% BF
		293	2 cups OAT BRAN FLAKES CEREAL, RTE
Notes:			
Meal Totals:	**Calories: 667**	**Carbs: 87g (52%)**	**Protein: 39g (23%) Fat: 19g (25%) Fluid: 34oz**
10:00 am	Snack	101	1 tablespoons ALMOND BUTTER, NO SALT
		120	1 muffin ENGLISH MUFFIN, 100% WHOLE WHEAT
		55	1 small APPLE W/SKIN, RAW
		0	16 fl oz WATER, DRINKING WATER, PURIFIED
Notes:			
Meal Totals:	**Calories: 276**	**Carbs: 41g (57%)**	**Protein: 8g (11%) Fat: 10g (33%) Fluid: 21oz**
12:00 pm	Lunch	176	20 crackers CRACKER, WHEAT THIN, BAKED
		151	2 pita BREAD, PITA, WHOLE WHEAT
		214	4 oz TURKEY BREAST, ROASTED
		0	16 fl oz WATER, DRINKING WATER, PURIFIED
		33	1 teaspoons MAYONNAISE, OLIVE OIL, ARTISAN
		8	2 oz TOMATO, RAW
		83	1 cups CARROT, BABY, RAW
		3	2 leaf LETTUCE, COS OR ROMAINE, RAW
Notes:			
Meal Totals:	**Calories: 668**	**Carbs: 59g (40%)**	**Protein: 42g (28%) Fat: 21g (32%) Fluid: 24oz**
03:00 pm	Snack	82	1/2 oz ALMOND, RAW
		179	6 oz YOGURT, FRUIT, LOW FAT
		61	1 large PEACH, RAW
		0	16 fl oz WATER, DRINKING WATER, PURIFIED
Notes:			
Meal Totals:	**Calories: 322**	**Carbs: 58g (61%)**	**Protein: 12g (15%) Fat: 9g (25%) Fluid: 27oz**
06:00 pm	Dinner	75	1 roll ROLL, DINNER, WHOLE WHEAT
		0	16 fl oz WATER, DRINKING WATER, PURIFIED
		621	CHICKEN VEGETABLE SOUP (TOTALS) (1.5 Servings)
Notes:			
Meal Totals:	**Calories: 696**	**Carbs: 87g (38%)**	**Protein: 66g (38%) Fat: 19g (24%) Fluid: 17oz**

Continued on next page ...

SLF Monthly Plan

Day 5

Day 5

Time	Meal Label	Calories	Meal Items
08:00 pm	Snack	180	2 bars GRANOLA BAR, OATS 'N HONEY
		102	1/2 cups COTTAGE CHEESE, 2% FAT
		0	8 fl oz WATER, DRINKING WATER, PURIFIED
		90	1 small BANANA, RAW
Notes:			
Meal Totals:	**Calories: 372**	**Carbs: 56g (59%)**	**Protein: 21g (22%) Fat: 8g (19%) Fluid: 16oz**

	Calories	Carbs	Protein	Fat	Fluid
Day 5 Totals:	**3001**	**360g (49%)**	**188g (25%)**	**86g (26%)**	**139oz**

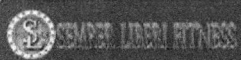
SEMPER LIBERI FITNESS

Become Free

Meal Plan
SLF Monthly Meal Plan

Prepared By: James Mullins
Email: semperliberifitness@gmail.com
Created: 10-11-2015

Day 6

Time	Meal Label	Calories	Meal Items
07:00 am	Breakfast	165	1 1/2 cups MILK, FLUID, PART SKIM, 1% BF
		61	1 large PEACH, RAW
		203	2 tablespoons ALMOND BUTTER, NO SALT
		0	16 fl oz WATER, DRINKING WATER, PURIFIED
		240	2 muffin ENGLISH MUFFIN, 100% WHOLE WHEAT
Notes:			
Meal Totals:	**Calories: 669**	**Carbs: 87g (50%)**	**Protein: 31g (18%) Fat: 25g (32%) Fluid: 33oz**
10:00 am	Snack	82	1/2 oz ALMOND, RAW
		114	1 3/8 cups BLUEBERRY, RAW
		0	16 fl oz WATER, DRINKING WATER, PURIFIED
		203	1 cups COTTAGE CHEESE, 2% FAT
Notes:			
Meal Totals:	**Calories: 399**	**Carbs: 40g (39%)**	**Protein: 35g (34%) Fat: 12g (26%) Fluid: 30oz**
12:00 pm	Lunch	621	CHICKEN VEGETABLE SOUP (TOTALS) (1.5 Servings)
		75	1 roll ROLL, DINNER, WHOLE WHEAT
		0	16 fl oz WATER, DRINKING WATER, PURIFIED
		35	1 teaspoons BUTTER
Notes:			
Meal Totals:	**Calories: 731**	**Carbs: 67g (36%)**	**Protein: 66g (36%) Fat: 23g (28%) Fluid: 18oz**
03:00 pm	Snack	224	12 toasts CRACKER, MELBA TOAST, WHEAT
		80	1 piece STRING CHEESE
		0	16 fl oz WATER, DRINKING WATER, PURIFIED
		55	1 small APPLE W/SKIN, RAW
Notes:			
Meal Totals:	**Calories: 359**	**Carbs: 62g (67%)**	**Protein: 15g (16%) Fat: 7g (17%) Fluid: 21oz**
06:00 pm	Dinner	216	1 cups BROWN RICE, LONG GRAIN, COOKED
		226	3/4 cups BEAN, BLACK, BOILED
		41	1 cups SPINACH, BOILED, NO SALT
		92	3 oz SALMON, ATLANTIC, WILD, BAKED OR BROILED
		0	16 fl oz WATER, DRINKING WATER, PURIFIED
Notes:			
Meal Totals:	**Calories: 575**	**Carbs: 93g (63%)**	**Protein: 38g (26%) Fat: 7g (11%) Fluid: 34oz**
08:00 pm	Snack	180	2 bars GRANOLA BAR, OATS 'N HONEY
		90	1 small BANANA, RAW
		0	8 fl oz WATER, DRINKING WATER, PURIFIED

Continued on next page ...

Day 6

Time	Meal Label	Calories	Meal Items		
Notes:					
	Meal Totals:	**Calories: 270**	**Carbs: 52g (74%)**	**Protein: 5g (7%) Fat: 6g (19%) Fluid: 12oz**	
		Calories	Carbs	Protein	Fat	Fluid
	Day 6 Totals:	**3003**	**401g (52%)**	**190g (25%)**	**80g (23%)**	**148oz**

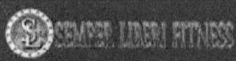
Meal Plan
SLF Monthly Meal Plan

Prepared By: **James Mullins**
Email: **semperliberifitness@gmail.com**
Created: **10-11-2015**

SLF Monthly Plan

Day 7

Day 7			
Time	Meal Label	Calories	Meal Items
07:00 am	Breakfast	35	1 teaspoons BUTTER
		179	6 oz YOGURT, FRUIT, LOW FAT
		0	16 fl oz WATER, DRINKING WATER, PURIFIED
		155	2 egg EGG, CHICKEN, WHOLE, HARD, BOILED
		90	1 small BANANA, RAW
		160	2 slice 100% WHOLE WHEAT BREAD
Notes:			
Meal Totals	Calories: 619	Carbs: 83g (54%)	Protein: 30g (19%) Fat: 19g (27%) Fluid: 28oz
10:00 am	Snack	80	1 piece STRING CHEESE
		150	6 toasts CRACKER, MELBA TOAST, WHEAT
		83	1 cups CARROT, BABY, RAW
		0	16 fl oz WATER, DRINKING WATER, PURIFIED
Notes:			
Meal Totals	Calories: 313	Carbs: 32g (54%)	Protein: 12g (20%) Fat: 7g (26%) Fluid: 17oz
12:00 pm	Lunch	340	2 wrap WRAP, 100% WHOLE WHEAT
		129	6 oz GRAPE, RAW
		120	4 oz ROAST BEEF LUNCHMEAT
		176	20 crackers CRACKER, WHEAT THIN, BAKED
		8	2 oz TOMATO, RAW
		2	16 fl oz ICED TEA, UNSWEETENED
		67	2 teaspoons MAYONNAISE, OLIVE OIL, ARTISAN
Notes:			
Meal Totals	Calories: 842	Carbs: 109g (52%)	Protein: 32g (15%) Fat: 31g (33%) Fluid: 25oz
03:00 pm	Snack	55	1 small APPLE W/SKIN, RAW
		180	2 bars GRANOLA BAR, OATS 'N HONEY
		0	16 fl oz WATER, DRINKING WATER, PURIFIED
Notes:			
Meal Totals	Calories: 235	Carbs: 44g (72%)	Protein: 4g (7%) Fat: 6g (22%) Fluid: 21oz
06:00 pm	Dinner	204	8 oz SWEET POTATO, BAKED, NO SALT
		151	2 roll ROLL, DINNER, WHOLE WHEAT
		225	5 oz CHICKEN, BROILER, BREAST, MEAT, ROASTED
		40	1 teaspoons OLIVE OIL, EXTRA VIRGIN
		39	1 cups KALE, BOILED, NO SALT
		0	16 fl oz WATER, DRINKING WATER, PURIFIED
Notes:			

Continued on next page...

SLF Monthly Plan

Day 7

Day 7			
Time	Meal Label	Calories	Meal Items
Meal Totals	Calories: 659	Carbs: 83g (49%)	Protein: 60g (35%) Fat: 12g (16%) Fluid: 33oz
08:00 pm	Snack	0	8 fl oz WATER, DRINKING WATER, PURIFIED
		203	1 cups COTTAGE CHEESE, 2% FAT
		81	1 pear PEAR, RAW
		41	1/4 oz ALMOND, RAW
Notes:			
Meal Totals	Calories: 325	Carbs: 30g (37%)	Protein: 34g (41%) Fat: 8g (22%) Fluid: 21oz

	Calories	Carbs	Protein	Fat	Fluid
Day 7 Totals:	2993	382g (52%)	172g (23%)	83g (25%)	145oz

Italian Chicken (totals) (serves 4)

Ingredients

- 4 dash Pepper, Black, Ground
- 2 teaspoons Oregano, Dried, Ground
- 2 clove Garlic, Raw
- 4 teaspoons Lemon Juice
- 2 tablespoons Olive Oil
- 16 oz Chicken, Breast W/o Skin, Raw

Instructions

Combine ingredients in a small bowl and place chicken breast in the bowl to marinate. Remember to turn it over occasionally. One hour before serving, heat oven to 450F. Line a baking sheet with foil, and put chicken on. Put pan in oven, reduce heat to 325F. Bake 35-45 minutes.

Chicken Vegetable Soup (totals) (serves 4)

Ingredients

- 2 tablespoons Vegetable Oil, Canola
- 2 medium Onion, Raw
- 2 cups Carrot, Raw
- 4 large Zucchini W/skin, Raw
- 2 tablespoons Parsley, Dried
- 2 teaspoons Oregano, Dried, Leaves
- 1/2 teaspoons Black Pepper, Ground
- 8 cups Vegetable Cooking Stock
- 16 oz Chicken Breast, Boneless, Roasted, Meat Only

Instructions

1. In a large saucepan, cook diced onion, zucchini and carrots in coconut oil until tender.
2. Season with pepper, oregano and parsley.
3. Add cooked chicken and vegetable stock.
4. Simmer over low heat for 15 minutes, stirring occasionally.

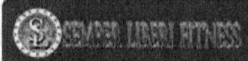
Meal Plan Shopping List

Category	Quantity	Item
Accompaniments	5 teaspoons	Mayonnaise, Olive Oil, Artisan	Spectrum
Beef	8 oz	Beef, Flank, Flank Steak, Lean, 0" Trim, Broiled
Beverages	7 1/4 cups	Milk, Fluid, Part Skim, 1% Bf
	32 fl oz	Iced Tea, Unsweetened	Generic
	568 fl oz	Water, Drinking Water, Purified
Bread	2 wrap	Wrap, 100% Whole Wheat	Sahara
	6 roll	Roll, Dinner, Whole Wheat
	6 slice	100% Whole Wheat Bread	Sara Lee
	7 muffin	English Muffin, 100% Whole Wheat	Thomas'
	8 pita	Bread, Pita, Whole Wheat
Cereal and Grain Products	2 cups	Oats, Rolled, Old Fashioned (oatmeal)	Quaker
	3 cups	Brown Rice, Long Grain, Cooked
	15 oz	Pasta, Macaroni Whole Wheat, Cooked
Cereals, Ready to Eat	4 cups	Oat Bran Flakes Cereal, Rte	Complete All Bran
Cookies & Crackers	58 toasts	Cracker, Melba Toast, Wheat
	80 crackers	Cracker, Wheat Thin, Baked	Nabisco
Dairy Products	4 large	Egg, Chicken, Hard-boiled
	4 teaspoons	Butter
	4 1/2 cups	Cottage Cheese, 2% Fat
	5 piece	String Cheese	Kraft
	7 egg	Egg, Chicken, Whole, Hard, Boiled
	26 oz	Yogurt, Fruit, Low Fat
Fats and Oils	5 1/2 teaspoons	Olive Oil, Extra Virgin	Bertolli
Finfish and Shellfish Products	3 oz	Salmon, Atlantic, Wild, Baked Or Broiled
	4 oz	Albacore Tuna In Water, Chunk White, Canned, Lower Sodium	Chicken of the Sea
	4 oz	Tilapia, Fresh	Wegmans
Fruits	4 large	Peach, Raw
	4 pear	Pear, Raw
	4 tablespoons	Cranberry, Dried, Sweetened
	4 3/8 cups	Blueberry, Raw
	5 small	Apple W/skin, Raw
	5 small	Banana, Raw
	18 oz	Grape, Raw
Ingredients	3 teaspoons	Balsamic Vinegar	Spectrum
Legumes	1 1/2 cups	Bean, Black, Boiled

Continued on next page...

Meal Plan Shopping List

Category	Quantity	Item
Nuts and Seeds	4 oz	Almond, Raw
	7 tablespoons	Almond Butter, No Salt
Poultry	9 oz	Turkey Breast, Roasted
	10 oz	Chicken, Broiler, Breast, Meat, Roasted
Sausages and Lunch Meats	4 oz	Roast Beef Lunchmeat	Hilshire Farm
Snacks	13 bars	Granola Bar, Oats 'n Honey	Nature Valley
Vegetables	1 cups	Broccoli, Boiled, No Salt
	1 cups	Zucchini W/skin, Boiled, No Salt
	2 cups	Kale, Boiled, No Salt
	2 cups	Spinach, Boiled, No Salt
	3 cups	Lettuce, Cos Or Romaine, Raw
	5 loaf	Lettuce, Cos Or Romaine, Raw
	9 3/4 cups	Carrot, Baby, Raw
	11 oz	Tomato, Raw
	16 oz	Sweet Potato, Baked, No Salt

Recipe Shopping List

Category	Quantity	Item
Beverages	4 teaspoons	Lemon Juice
Fats and Oils	2 tablespoons	Olive Oil
	2 tablespoons	Vegetable Oil, Canola
Poultry	16 oz	Chicken Breast, Boneless, Roasted, Meat Only
	16 oz	Chicken, Breast W/o Skin, Raw
Soup	8 cups	Vegetable Cooking Stock	Imagine
Spices	1/2 teaspoons	Black Pepper, Ground	McCormick/Schilling
	2 tablespoons	Parsley, Dried
	2 teaspoons	Oregano, Dried, Ground
	2 teaspoons	Oregano, Dried, Leaves
	4 dash	Pepper, Black, Ground
Vegetables	2 clove	Garlic, Raw
	2 cups	Carrot, Raw
	2 medium	Onion, Raw
	4 large	Zucchini W/skin, Raw

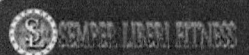

Portion Guide

Knowing exactly how much is on your plate can be tricky. Visualizing tablespoons, ounces, and cups of food isn't easy, which makes dishing out correct serving sizes a challenge. We've created the comparisons below as an easy guideline to help calculate proper portion sizes.

Basic Guidelines

Golf Ball	Tennis Ball	Computer Mouse	Baseball	Rounded Handful
¼ cup 1 oz 2 tbsp	⅓ cup	½ cup	1 cup	⅓ cup 1 oz dried goods

Hockey Puck	Matchbox	Deck of Cards	Thin Paperback Book	Thumb
3 oz muffin or biscuit	1 oz serving of meat	3 oz of chicken, meat, or fish	8 oz serving of meat	1 tsp

Poker Chip	Shot Glass	CD	3 Dice	Kids' School Milk Carton
1 tbsp	1 oz 2 tbsp	1 slice of bread 1 oz lunch meat	1 ½ oz cheese	8 oz drink

Useful Examples

Bread & Grains

1 cup of cereal = 1 baseball
½ cup cooked rice = computer mouse
½ cup cooked paste = computer mouse
1 slice of bread = CD
3 cups of popcorn = 3 baseballs

Fruits & Vegetables

½ cup grapes = about 16 grapes
1 cup of strawberries = about 12 berries
1 cup of salad greens = 1 baseball
1 cup cooked vegetables = 1 baseball
1 baked potato = computer mouse

Meats, Fish & Nuts

3 oz lean meat or poultry = deck of cards
3 oz tofu = deck of cards
2 tbsp peanut butter = golf ball
¼ cup almonds = about 23 almonds
¼ cup pistachios = about 24 pistachios

Dairy & Cheese

1 ½ oz cheese = stacked dice
1 cup yogurt = baseball
½ cup ice cream = computer mouse

Fats & Oils

1 tbsp butter or spread = poker chip
1 tbsp salad dressing = poker chip
1 tbsp oil or mayonnaise = poker chip

Sweets & Treats

1 slice cake = deck of cards
1 cookie = about 2 poker chips
1 piece of chocolate = matchbox

After you have chosen a training program that you will enjoy and a nutrition program that is aligned with your BMR, you are ready to begin your journey. All you have to do to progress is follow the training plans and stick to your meal plan. With these tools, you are on the path to success.

The training plans are all set for short-term goals, and the meal plans are set up for a week. These are enough tools for you to get started and make sure the training plans are something you enjoy and that the meal plan is something that you can follow.

The benefits of having this various meal and training plans are that it allows you to try different things each week. You can try a circuit training plan for a week, a strength program for a week and then a fat burning program. This allows you to mix it up and try some different things until you find the program that you love the most. At that point, you can then seek out resources to begin that program long term.

With the nutrition programs, you have similar variability. You can choose the program for your Basal Metabolic Rate(BMR) and follow it for a week. You can then use the other programs and add or subtract foods as needed to meet your caloric needs.

The whole purpose of our programs is to help with flexibility and make sure you have the right program for you. With a coach to guide you it is easier to learn and adjust to make sure you get the best results but adjusting these programs can be done on your own. There are many different foods and food choices listed and with the shopping guides, calorie values, and portion guide you have all of the tools to adjust as needed to get foods you love and healthy results.

Once again, if you want to get individualized training programs and meals plans that allow you to substitute your foods via a smartphone app or software, we have these options available. They are much more in depth and have more flexibility.

My goal when I began Semper Liberi was to make sure that I give a positive and supportive atmosphere to anyone who is looking to improve their health and their life. I knew that I wanted to share my personal experiences with others as a way to extend that support to others.

I know how hard getting results was for me, and I also know the struggles of finding something that will get you in shape that you love and enjoy. With the programs and resources, I have shared, you should be well on your way to finding the best path for you.

Conclusion

"Create a definite plan for carrying out your desire and begin at once, whether you ready or not, to put this plan into action."

- Napoleon Hill

I hope I the future I can continue to share information like this with you. I want to get more in-depth with some of the programs and give you some step by step guides to follow in each, but that will come later.

For now, I will close with trying to make you as comfortable as possible in beginning a program. People want you to succeed and that we have many resources available to support you. We have Facebook groups to support you, and our membership site is an excellent place to make sure you have all the support you need to reach your goals. You can always reach out to me, and I will help you in the best way that I can.

Remember, though, all we can do is offer support and give you the resources and tools to succeed. The work is up to you. You have to take action. As Tony Robbins says "The path to success is to take massive, determined action." So, go ahead, choose a program, get your meal plan, and begin your start your journey today. **You can do it; I know you can!**

www.ingramcontent.com/pod-product-compliance
Lightning Source LLC
Chambersburg PA
CBHW060332290526
45793CB00003B/604